THE

CANCER

COMPANION

About the author

Dr Toni Lindsay is a qualified Clinical and Health Psychologist who has been working with both adults and adolescents for over ten years. She works at Chris O'Brien Lifehouse in the Oncology department, and has a special interest in the care of adolescents and young adults with cancer. She is an AHPRA-approved supervisor and works predominantly from an Acceptance and Commitment Therapy framework.

THE
CANCER
COMPANION

How to navigate your
way from diagnosis
to treatment and beyond

Dr TONI LINDSAY

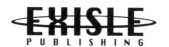

EXISLE
PUBLISHING

First published 2021

Exisle Publishing Pty Ltd
PO Box 864, Chatswood, NSW 2057, Australia
226 High Street, Dunedin, 9016, New Zealand
www.exislepublishing.com

A CiP record for this book is available from the National Library of Australia.

ISBN 978-1-925820-80-5

Designed by Mark Thacker
Typeset in Minion Pro regular 10.75 on 14.5pt
Printed in China

This book uses paper sourced under ISO 14001 guidelines from well-managed forests and other controlled sources.

10 9 8 7 6 5 4 3 2 1

To all the people who
have shared their stories.

Contents

Part 4: The psychology part: How can you manage all of this?

Welcome

If you have picked up this book it's likely that you or someone in your world has been diagnosed with something.

It might be something that the doctors are saying is okay and will be simple to fix. Or they may be saying the opposite, that it is something that can't be fixed. Or somewhere in between. Regardless, it's likely you are feeling a bunch of things you might not have felt before.

This might look like fear, or terror or anger. Or it might be nothing, with no thoughts in your mind at all, a quiet that you know can't last. Or it might be loud and thunderous, with more thoughts than you can pay attention to all zooming from corner to corner in your brain. Or you might feel relieved that the thing you have been worried about for so long finally has a name and a plan. Or you might be just hoping and pretending all of this will go away, and by keeping busy the reality will slip off back to where it came from, unnoticed.

Whichever of these it is (or it might be others, or a combination of all of them), you aren't going mad.

This book isn't meant to fix any of these things — these things that are coming up for you are meant to be there. And it isn't likely that you will be able to get rid of them or 'fix' them. It's likely that nothing like this has ever happened before, so it makes sense that the way you think and feel about it will be different to how you have thought about things in the past.

For now, it's about trying to make sense of what is happening in your head, and the heads of the people around you, when your world is suddenly turned upside down.

The thoughts in this book aren't from my experience. They are the collective wisdom and worries of thousands of people with cancer and their families who have shared some of their emotional experiences with me. This book will step you through the main stages and concerns that people have during their cancer experiences. Some people will be surrounded by lots of family and friends, while others may feel quite isolated. Either way, many of my patients talk about feeling that no one understands what they are going through. Hopefully, this book will provide some voices that offer some shared experience and ideas about how to navigate your way through the difficult times.

Like most books, it's best not to read ahead. It's likely that your brain is already projecting forward into an uncertain future and panicking, with loads of thoughts about what might happen next. You might even be mourning the loss of some of your future. If you read too far ahead — or even, for that matter, *think* too far ahead — that feeling of overwhelm is likely to come in like an unexpected wave, knocking you off your feet and dumping you on the shore. Instead, reminding yourself of where you are right now, in this moment, is helpful. You know what is happening right now. You can make decisions about right now. That's much harder for the next 24 hours, two days or year. I am talking about being focused on the next moment, or the next hour, no further out than that. You can do something in the here and now. Even if what you are focused on is a very small thing, it is likely to feel helpful. Lots of the things we will talk about in this book are about helping you get through lots of little moments rather than big, nebulous things that are too huge to even try to make sense of.

The book is broken into small chapters that you can hopefully absorb in bite-sized chunks. If you read it once and it doesn't make sense, come back to it later. People move through all this at different times, so some information might not be applicable to you, or it might not be the right time for you. I have tried to order the information logically, based on how things might progress emotionally for people. But if everyone was able to do this all the same way it would be easy to navigate. So I am willing to bet at least once or twice you will read some of this and it won't be the right fit, won't make sense or you might just think it's rubbish. That is okay too.

In this book, you will find some quotes and stories from people. These are based on the experiences of lots of people I have met over the years, and any identifying details have been removed. Hopefully, there will be things in their stories that will help you in navigating your own story. Sometimes it can be really comforting to know you aren't alone in something.

The first three parts of the book talk about the stages of cancer — being diagnosed and starting treatment, finishing treatment, and managing advanced disease. Part 4 of the book is about the psychological things you can do to help you navigate through these. I have made sure to cross-reference, so if, for instance, we are talking about managing thoughts about chemotherapy, I will direct you to the chapter where you can learn some strategies to help with this.

Tips for carers

It is important to note that it is not only the person with the disease who is impacted by cancer. For every patient, there are generally at least a couple of people travelling along with them and trying to make sense of this too. So, throughout the book, you will find some helpful tips for carers. These might be about how to better meet the needs of the person who is unwell, or they might be about the carer's own feelings.

Some important concepts we'll talk about in the book

Part of what makes cancer challenging is that people sometimes try to use strategies that have worked to manage thoughts and worries in the past, but find they don't work with these new cancer worries. This is largely because the worries are different.

Most people find they worry about things that fit into two categories: worries that are fixable, and worries that are quite irrational (there are some others, but let's focus on these two for now). When a worry is fixable — it might be a problem or something you can think through logically — our brain does pretty well with them. We are naturally good problem solvers and can generally get to a place where we can make sense of whatever is troubling us. The other type of worry is the one where we get caught up in something we recognize is probably a bit irrational (this doesn't stop us getting caught up in it, though). It might be about other people, or thoughts about ourselves; for instance, when we convince ourselves that we said something stupid at lunch and weren't as funny as we thought. For some people, these kinds of thoughts might be fleeting, but others will kick them around and around in their minds. To get rid of these thoughts it's sometimes helpful to tell yourself that they are ridiculous, or do something to distract yourself. And for these types of thoughts you may have found this works really well.

But for thoughts about the cancer, these things probably won't work as well. For some practical things — like having to decide between two types of treatment — problem-solving your way through will work really well. For these kinds of thoughts, we will talk about strategies that look at challenging the thought and examining its helpfulness. (Within psychology land we call these strategies Cognitive Behaviour Therapy (CBT). Both types of strategies that we'll talk about in this book — CBT and Acceptance and Commitment Therapy, or ACT — are cognitive therapies; that is, they are concerned with the way we think.) But those other thoughts — like the ones around what is going to happen in the future, or fears about the cancer coming back — aren't likely to respond to this stuff. Because the worries about cancer are different.

Cancer worries don't tend to have an answer. No one can tell you for certain what is going to happen in the future, and even if you are told that your treatment is finished and all is okay, you are likely to have worries about the cancer coming back. People can very clearly tell me that they know things will probably be okay, but they can't stop worrying about it. This isn't something that problem-solving will work for, or something you can tell yourself not to worry about. And you can't convince yourself you are thinking irrationally. Actually, for these kinds of thoughts, usually trying not to think about them doesn't work at all. They will just appear somewhere else (usually at 3 a.m.) because they are different types of worries. Distraction might work a little bit, but usually in a temporary way.

Acceptance and Commitment Therapy

So, I would like to borrow some ideas from a type of therapy called Acceptance and Commitment Therapy, or ACT for short (if you are interested to read further, see the References list on p. 208). The main premise of ACT is that, as human beings, we will experience difficult things and challenges to our sense of existence. We can fight against these things, or we can learn to manage what it means to have these things present in our lives. Instead of trying to get rid of thoughts and difficult feelings, and pushing them away, we learn how to allow them to be present in our lives. It takes incredible amounts of energy to try to get rid of anything difficult or unpleasant that comes into our minds.

I would like you to do an experiment. When you have read this, I would like you to set a timer on your phone for two minutes and close your eyes. Until you hear the timer go off, I want you to stop thinking. I want you to turn off the thought machine and have nothing in your mind.

How did you go?

I am willing to bet that I set you an almost impossible task. You might have been able to do it for a couple of seconds, but I doubt you managed a couple of minutes (I'm happy to be proven wrong). But I am hoping that what you noticed is that by doing this you are trying to stop your brain doing its job. Our mind thinks constantly — while we are eating and sleeping and talking. If we try to stop it thinking, we are stopping it doing its job.

So why would we try to stop our brain worrying about things that feel so important, like cancer?

It doesn't make much sense that you could simply not think about the cancer, or what might happen next. And it doesn't seem that it would be helpful for your brain to never think about these things ever again.

Instead, in this book I talk a lot about the idea of allowing these thoughts to be present and just noticing them. By this, I don't mean trying to push them out of your mind or getting rid of them. I mean that, when these difficult thoughts come up, just tell yourself that it is okay they are there, and notice what happens in your body and how you feel when they are present.

This might feel really unnatural. We have changed the game, right? You have probably been trying to get rid of any difficult thoughts your entire life. And now we are going to let them be there, and often expect them to be there. And think about it being okay that they are there (and almost expecting them to be!).

When thoughts turn up in our mind it is hard to believe they might not be true. It might be that you do have many thoughts that are accurate, but there will also be many that aren't. The other important premise in changing the way we think about thinking is recognizing that the things that show up in our mind are just thoughts. When they are swirling around in your mind it's hard to believe that they aren't 100 per cent accurate, particularly when they feel so real. But the thoughts are a result of your brain doing a job. They aren't predictive or informing or sometimes even accurate — they are just thoughts.

It is helpful thing to remind yourself of this (and even tell yourself) when the thoughts are loud and convincing you how terrible all of this is. Or at 3 a.m. when the night is quiet and you are terrified, and the thoughts keep coming.

They are just thoughts.

And they are thoughts that we expect to appear. Cancer is a really tricky character. It fills us with uncertainty and worry about the future, and often tells us that we aren't going to be okay. So in this situation it makes sense that we might expect some difficult thoughts and anxieties to come up, right? In fact, if they didn't turn up that would be even more perplexing. Can you imagine your mind with absolutely no thoughts?

Just remember, it's your brain doing its job. Cancer is likely to bring lots of these things up, and it's okay that they arrive. They are just thoughts, and we will work out what to do with them.

By the way, this will also work for any other thoughts in your life, not just the cancer ones.

So, enough about that. Let's just get on and talk about it.

Part 1

On treatment

Jane is 48 years old and is used to juggling things. She has a very successful career as a lawyer in a big inner city firm, and has a husband, David, and two kids, Molly and Ethan, who are seven and nine respectively. Jane and David have a strong group of friends they've known since university, as well as a bunch of people they have got to know in their local area with kids the same age as theirs. They like to go on holidays, and have a trip planned to the Gold Coast in a couple of weeks, because Molly is finally tall enough to go on the rides at the theme parks.

For the past couple of months Jane has been feeling tired. Well, she always feels tired, but she has felt more tired than normal. She has also been bloated. Not so much that other people would notice it, but when she eats she feels uncomfortable. She had gone to the GP, who suggested Jane go for a scan, but she hadn't managed to get the time to do it.

One day while she was waiting for Molly at soccer practice, Jane felt a sharp stabbing pain in her abdomen. She thought it would go away, but that night she ended up in the emergency department. She was given lots of scans and tests, but she knew when the doctor appeared in the early hours of the morning at the end of her bed that the news wasn't good. She had a big tumour in her ovary and they were worried about something in her liver. The doctor told Jane other things, but she couldn't remember what they were, and if she is honest, she didn't take in much information for the rest of the night, or the next day, with lots of doctors and surgeons coming to talk to her. She was taken for surgery a couple of days later, and it was confirmed: she had ovarian cancer.

David, Jane's husband, went into planning mode, scouring the internet looking for as much information as he could about ovarian cancer and possible treatments. Every time he saw one of the doctors he had lots and lots of questions, but he seemed to find that the more questions he asked, the more muddled things got in his head, and the more anxious he got. Jane didn't really feel anything at all. She knew it was happening, and she knew it couldn't be good, but she couldn't make herself think about it anymore than that. It was almost as if it didn't feel real.

Before Jane went for the surgery she was a little nervous, but it wasn't until she saw the scar across her stomach, just above where she had the caesarean scar from when she had Molly, that she started to make sense of it. Even then, it felt like a blur that she didn't quite know what to do with. She knew that she should tell people, and talk with the kids, but all she wanted to do was watch Netflix. She had told work that she would be away, but was still hoping that perhaps she would be back in a couple of weeks.

As the days went on, Jane and David were getting grumpy at each other, and neither knew what to do. When the doctor told them Jane would need to have chemotherapy, she sent a text message to all her friends and family, and was of course inundated with offers of support. There were people who started calling her many times a day, and then there were people she heard nothing from, which made her feel a combination of anger and sadness. Some people, who Jane thought would be the most helpful when something bad happened, turned out to be not very helpful at all.

When Jane got home from the hospital, she and David sat down with the kids and told them that she was sick, but didn't want to use the word cancer. There had been some other kids in their classes with parents who had cancer, and she didn't want them to be worried. And they weren't. They just kept going to school and playing with their friends in the same way they always did. They had casseroles and spaghetti bolognese delivered almost every day by different friends. Jane felt completely overwhelmed by the support.

While Jane recovered, she knew she should be sorting things out. She had been told that the treatment was pretty difficult, so she knew she should organize things for the kids and David in case she wasn't well enough to do what she normally did. She thought a lot about what she needed to do, but felt too exhausted to do any of it. She had tried to keep things as normal as possible, but found she wasn't able to focus and pay attention very well. She had tried to do some work from home but couldn't manage it. Jane started to panic that she would always be like this. She couldn't sleep, and when she lay in bed at night thoughts popped into her head that she couldn't bear to think about. She was scared, and she was anxious, but she felt like she couldn't tell anyone, because Jane was always able to manage things. Instead, she smiled, told people she was doing well, and spent lots of her time worrying about things when no one was looking.

1.

And then it was cancer ...

The news hit me with a thud. And then my ears felt like they
were ringing for days. I couldn't hear or make sense of a
word anyone was saying. And then it became clear, the words
smashing around in my head had meaning. I had cancer.
Katrina, 42 years old

I often think about the way that people describe the moment of being diagnosed as a bit of a vortex, where the world seems to speed up and slow
down at the same time. If this has happened to you recently, I suspect this
feeling will be quite close to the surface for you.

Research has shown that after people hear the word 'cancer' they don't
hear anything else in the consultation, and it will often take several appointments with their doctors to start to make sense of what they are hearing.
The way people manage this will be different from person to person; but
most people, as with any other shocking bad news, are likely to feel quite
numb and disconnected to start with.

In my practice I often talk about the '72-hour window' or the time it takes to process this kind of information. For the first couple of days after people receive such information they usually aren't able to process it, not in any real way. They are likely to cry, be shocked, distressed, angry, sad, insulated and sombre or, even more likely, a combination of all these things. It may also be at this time that things like sleep, appetite and attention span change temporarily, with people feeling like they just want to be distracted and a bit disconnected from what is going on. Grief and the processing of life events rarely happen in any type of linear way, so people will oscillate through some or all of these emotions, often shifting from one to the other within moments or hours.

At these times, it is about moving through the emotions and letting them be rather than trying to do anything else. This process is part of your brain doing its work rather than anything to be worried about. But it will feel different to how you generally feel. Take the time you need to make sense of whatever you need to make sense of. This might happen multiple times through the cancer process, not just at the beginning — it might happen if you are given new information about the next lot of treatment, or a particular plan, or when you finish treatment, or if your cancer returns. And each time this happens it will feel as disconcerting and unfamiliar as the last. It's worth reminding yourself that this is what is meant to happen, and it will come to an end.

> I kept expecting that I would do something or feel something.
> Instead I just watched movie after movie and didn't think
> about it at all.
> Angelo, 56 years old

After the 72-hour window you are likely to have some more clarity of thought, and the shock will have subsided somewhat. This is also the time in cancer land where you may be more likely to have a bit of a plan forming for what happens next. This might be about having a treatment plan, or a discussion about further review by other people. This might be the time when your brain goes into practical and planning mode, which is one of the things that will largely help you manage through the next months of treatment, or whatever might come next. This is the time when, instead of being completely overwhelmed by the idea of uncertainty and panic, your brain will help you by shifting towards thoughts about how to navigate the next steps.

Behind the scenes

When someone is diagnosed it might initially feel like there is not much happening — perhaps they are getting sent for lots of scans and tests, and it might feel like an eternity between appointments where there is information being given.

Patients tell me that the time when it feels like nothing is happening is actually the time when lots of things are happening — you might just not know about them. At many hospitals and for most cancers there will be a group of people who will get together and talk about what is going to happen next for you. This is called a Multidisciplinary Team (or the MDT). This group usually includes oncologists, surgeons, pathologists, radiation oncologists, specialist nurses and psychosocial members. A member of the team (usually the person you have been referred to) will take your case to the meeting and seek the opinions of the others to ensure your treatment plan takes everything into account, and that all aspects of making sure you get the most effective treatment are covered off.

So although it feels like nothing is happening and you might even be worried they have forgotten about you, it's much more likely that a plan is being discussed and organized.

I just felt so desperate for someone to tell me it would all be okay, I was reading everything I could find. In the end, I realized all it was doing was making me realize that I wouldn't find an answer.

Liz, 50 years old

Beware of Dr Google: navigating through information

This can be the time when people start researching things like crazy, and I tell you, Dr Google has quite a lot to answer for.

We like to have answers and certainty, and you have just found yourself in the biggest pile of uncertainty you have likely ever encountered. Your brain will be flooded with thoughts about the future and what is going to happen next. I suspect thoughts and worries about whether you are going to die have started to be very present. So it makes perfect sense that in this uncertainty you would seek answers, right? And who can provide the answers? The internet. There are many difficulties with this, but here are the main issues:

Counterintuitively, the information on the internet about cancer and its treatments is often quite out of date.

The information you find isn't likely to be relevant to you, as cancer and its treatments are so individual, based on factors that your doctors and treating teams will take into account and that you might not even be aware of.

As a general rule, people don't talk about how great things are going when they talk about cancer on the internet. In all likelihood you will find yourself presented with a bunch of stories and experiences that are not representative of most people, and skewed very much towards how bad things can be.

If you put any cancer type and the words 'survival' into Google, it is likely that within the first pages and results, you will be presented concurrently with the word 'death'. This is in no way representative of your actual survival statistics.

When people go searching for answers to reassure their brains, they actually start to spin out more, a bit like a car stuck in the mud trying to get traction with its back wheels. So just like the car stuck in the mud, instead of trying to get out, you might be better off stopping and waiting for help to arrive. In the instance of cancer, that help is likely to be from your treating team, who will tell you what you need to know and give you a plan.

Write down your questions

Just after you get the news about the cancer (or whatever other information you might be trying to process) and before treatment starts, it is likely you will have lots of questions and worries. People tend to have many questions for their doctors between appointments, but then forget them the second they are sitting in the room; they then leave the consultation kicking themselves that they didn't get the information they needed.

In order to manage this, the simplest thing to do is to write some questions down before you go to your appointment and take some paper to write down the answers. Some doctors might be happy for you to record the consults so that you can listen back later, in case you miss the information. Also, if you can, take someone with you; they will probably miss some of the info as well, but at least with multiple sets of ears in the room the chance that most of the important stuff will be heard will increase.

The ways in which people process information and manage the time before starting treatment will look really different. It is about finding the way that makes the most sense for you. Some people manage by thinking endlessly about the cancer and what might happen next for them. But others might completely disconnect and appear not to be thinking about it at all. You might fall somewhere in between these two extremes, or it might change over time. In most cases, even if it appears that you aren't thinking about it, you probably will be thinking about it, rolling it around in the background of your brain without you realizing. Lots of people around you are likely to have ideas about what you should be doing, but I would say it is worth listening to your own brain and body on this one.

And if you feel as if you are freaking out and don't know which way is up, that is okay too.

TIPS FOR CARERS:
Becoming a carer

I imagine it is pretty unlikely you thought much about what it would mean to be caring for someone with cancer until it happened. And it can be a really scary place. Lots of the carers I talk with tell me they feel really confused about how they feel about their role. They will generally tell me very quickly (and honestly) that they would not consider doing anything else other than being there and helping their person who is unwell. They will do anything they can to make sure their person is doing as well as they can, and that they are making it as easy as possible on them.

The other side of this equation, though, is that caring comes at a cost to the person doing it. So since the diagnosis, it's likely you have felt some combination of the following:

- **anxious and overwhelmed**
- **worried about the future (both of the person who is unwell, and your own)**
- **relieved at having a plan**
- **unable to sleep, or finding you have more worries in your mind than normal**
- **numb and empty**
- **scared**
- **guilty at thoughts you might be having**
- **irritable and grumpy at the person you are caring for**
- **distracted and unable to focus**
- **frustrated**
- **thankful for the small things**
- **thinking about your own mortality.**

This, by the way, is not an exhaustive list. If you have felt things that aren't on this list, that is okay too!

The most important part of being a carer is working out what you need to keep **you** going. If you are exhausted and burnt out, it's not likely that you will be able to do any of the caring stuff. So, given that you don't know how long this carer journey is going to be, it's about the old adage of preparing for a marathon not a sprint. It's keeping on doing the small things in your world that make a big difference — getting to the gym a couple of times a week, catching up with friends, talking about things that aren't related to the cancer. If you keep these things ticking along, it helps to make sure that the fuel tank is always closer to full than empty.

2.

Normal

I just keep waiting for it all to be normal again — and it feels like it might never be. I just never realized how important all of the pieces of my pre-cancer life felt.

Fatima, 38 years old

You probably have a picture of what your normal is. And there is a reasonable chance that as a result of being diagnosed this will feel very different.

'Normal' is a word psychologists tend to shy away from — for many reasons, not the least of which is that we don't have a very good measure of it.

The concept of normal becomes more complex in the world of cancer and or chronic diseases. When people come into cancer land it is often unexpected, and they find themselves in a time of turbulence. When this happens, the concept of feeling normal might feel very distant, as plans and day-to-day activities shift and change. The world that was very boring and predictable last week can look entirely different in the weeks following a diagnosis. Often the things that take up blocks of time in people's lives disappear (like work, for instance) and from the outside looking in, their worlds could not look more changed. But perhaps that is now normal?

At the initial stage of diagnosis, your time is likely spent moving between medical appointments and procedures, with little time for anything else. You may have had to stay in hospital for a long time, which means that day-to-day normality will look entirely different. As a result, the craving for reconnecting with what your days looked like before cancer might start to creep in. You might even be having thoughts about how you could possibly manage this for the time the doctors are telling you treatment will take.

When treatment begins

When treatment starts, people can be unsettled and unsure about what to do with themselves. Will they be sick? Will they be able to work? Will they be able to keep doing what they want to do? If you ask doctors these questions they might answer in a vague way to start with, and this is not because they are being obtuse. For every treatment, there are some people who will fly through it, having almost no side effects, and they might suspect their doctors are not giving them the right treatment or medications. At the other end, there will be people who will be so unwell they cannot bear the thought of having any more. Although they may have some clues, the doctors don't know at the outset which one of those people you are going to be, and in all likelihood, like most people, you will be somewhere in the middle.

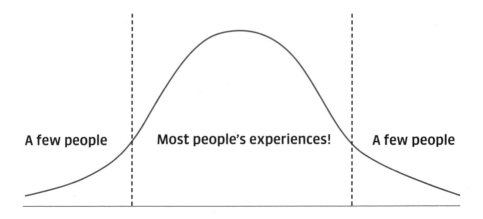

A few people   Most people's experiences!   A few people

But thinking about the concept of normal, it begs the question: how can you be normal if you don't know what the treatment is going to do to you? Perhaps that is normal.

Survival instinct

Human beings are resilient creatures. One of the most powerful instincts we have is to survive — this has allowed us to make our way through some pretty intense times in our history, and it will also help you now. Often the first thing people say to me when I ask them about what treatment they might be willing to accept or what they are going to do next is very simply: 'I will just do whatever I need to do.'

That is our survival instinct coming into play. It will allow you to make decisions, process information and work with things in a way you might not have thought about before. But now the stakes are probably a bit higher. The survival instinct is here to help you. It might mean, though, that some other things feel less important, or trivial. That's okay. One of the things the instinct can provide you with is the ability to focus on what needs to be the focus right now.

Keeping yourself grounded

It is tempting when entering the gates of cancer land to stop doing everything you were doing before. It even makes sense. How can you keep doing all these things that probably don't feel like they matter very much right now? When contrasted with something as huge as being diagnosed with cancer, there is a reasonable chance that mundane things like going to the shops and walking the dog will not feel very important. Except these are probably the kinds of things that will get you through all of this and make it feel a bit more manageable (just a bit).

In one of the many things that will feel counterintuitive about cancer, the more you keep doing the things that keep you grounded, give you a sense of routine, and of meaning and purpose, the more settled and okay you are likely to feel during the process. Without anything outside of your illness and treatment to focus on, you are likely to feel miserable (as in really miserable) within weeks. Having these other things in your life gives you something to focus on and look forward to, and can often provide some structure in a world that can very quickly lose all of the things that would normally provide it.

There are a few caveats to this, of course.

- There is a balance between helpful and harmful in the cancer setting (that is a little twitchier than before). What I mean by this is that if something feels nourishing and helpful, even if it is stressful at times, then it is probably worth doing. For instance, if picking up the kids from school every day means you can have some social contact and feel good for making the effort even when you physically feel terrible, then it is probably a good thing. But if you start feeling anxious and worried from the time the kids leave the house about going to get them, and it feels completely overwhelming, then it might not be worth it, and perhaps this is one of the activities that someone else can help you with.

- Sometimes during cancer and treatment, you won't feel like doing anything. At all. This is also okay, but it's best to check in about why you aren't wanting to do anything. Is it because you are really sick or in lots of pain (this is an okay reason)? Or do you just feel like you can't be bothered (a less okay reason)? One of the tricky things about motivation is that the less you do, the less you want to do, and so when people haven't been doing very much they can quickly become overwhelmed doing anything. In this case, the best thing to do is to start small — and I mean really small. If you would normally be able to do a whole basket of ironing, maybe start with two shirts. Or if you normally walk for 5 kilometres each Sunday maybe start with doing a smaller ten-minute walk. In all likelihood, when you start you will keep going, but with a brain that is fighting you on all of these things, the smaller the steps the better. We will talk about this lots more as we move through this process!

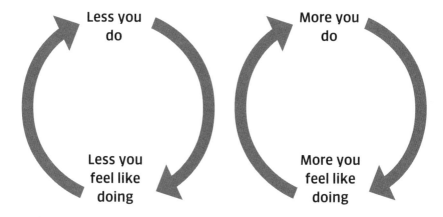

- There might be lots of pressure from the people around you, and in your wider circle, who will tell you what they think is the best thing for you to do. It's easy to get caught up in this advice (which is generally well meaning) and then become completely overwhelmed by it. If this starts to happen, step back for a bit and ask yourself: what is the stuff that is really important to you, and what is the stuff that you are doing because someone told you that you should? This should sort out most of these things, but if not, a good rule of thumb is to do the things that make you feel good first and then manage the rest later. I understand that just because cancer is around the rest of the world hasn't stopped, so not everything you do will be pleasant or meaningful; but some of the things that are not normally meaningful might start to feel like it in the context of everything that is going on. For instance, all of a sudden walking the dog in the sunshine might not feel like 'another thing that has to be done' — rather, it might feel very nourishing and revitalizing.
- You know yourself and your body better than anyone. If it is telling you to rest, then resting is okay.

We will talk about our good friend normal many times through the book. But just remember, normal is wherever you are right now. It just happens that this normal you sit in at the moment is likely to be different from where you have been before.

TIPS FOR CARERS:
What do you and the person you are caring for need?

The person you are caring for might show a bunch of different reactions at different times.

For instance, they might be:

- **distant and quiet while they try to process information**
- **talkative and wanting to work through every possible scenario with you**
- **focused on planning for the future and want to engage you in things like doing wills, estate planning, talking about finances or asking you to be their power of attorney**
- **appear that they aren't processing anything at all, and to you it might seem as if they aren't talking or thinking about the cancer at all.**

Each of these reactions is completely normal, but might require different responses from you as the carer.

If the person you are caring for is not engaging with you at all, this might make you feel very uncomfortable and you may feel as if you are not doing anything at all that feels helpful. If this is the case, then following their lead is probably the best option. Trying to force them into talking will likely frustrate them and exacerbate your sense of not being able to help. If they need to talk, they will talk eventually — it might just be after they have had some time to process what they need to think about. Being around and caring, without providing too much pressure, is probably the most helpful thing you can do.

Conversely, though, if your person wants to communicate about some of the things above, and you are comfortable in engaging with this, then it might be fine. However, for some people I speak to, the difficulty comes when there is a mismatch — for instance, if the patient wants to talk about everything but the carer feels completely overwhelmed when this happens. Or if you as the carer feel you are being forced to talk about things you don't feel comfortable talking about (this is particularly true if patients want to talk about death or financial matters that the carer doesn't want to talk about).

The key to managing this is usually to spell out what you need. For example, something like: 'This cancer thing has been really tough to process. I have noticed that it seems like we are managing it differently. At the moment I feel like it's really important for me to talk, but I don't think that feels helpful for you. What do you need from me?'

If you feel like you need extra support, it might be helpful to tap into a broader network who might be able to give you what you need, so that you are then able to support your person in the way they need.

3.

Finding your purpose and meaning:
part 1

And then all of a sudden everything about me had disappeared, and all I was, was this bloody cancer.
John, 60 years old

As mentioned earlier in the book, the idea of having purpose and meaning while undergoing treatment is incredibly important. For us to get out of bed in the mornings, even before cancer, there is invariably a need to have some aspects of our lives which feel meaningful for us. This meaning looks different for everyone, and will come in lots of shapes and sizes; sometimes what you find meaningful, the people around you will find much less so.

You might be reading this right now, thinking you don't know what the meaning is in your life. That's okay. Often these things aren't obvious, or they aren't things people think about until they are not there anymore.

Some of the things that give meaning do so for multiple reasons. For instance, with something like work, the actual work you do might feel meaningful and important, but the actual process of working can be meaningful in itself, in the sense that it makes you wake up in the mornings, go to work, behave in certain ways, have structure, etc. Similarly, people often identify their role with their family and friends as being meaningful, but might struggle to pinpoint what it is about that role that feels important. It might be to do with the relationship you have, it might be as your role as helper, or even the way you feel when you do things for people who are important to you.

For many people, the difficulty with the cancer process is that the things that generally help bolster them through life and give meaning and purpose may disappear temporarily (or in some cases permanently), and they may find themselves lost and for the first time having to think about these kinds of things. What further complicates it is that thinking about this is hard going sometimes, and people are often faced with doing so at a time when they have limited energy and capacity because of cancer treatments or other physical difficulties.

Yet another challenge in the cancer space is that there is a lie we have been sold. For a long time, a mythology has been built around cancer as being a gateway to epiphanies about the meaning of life, as well as a reason that people change everything about their lives. Now don't get me wrong, most people will experience a version of this, but it generally doesn't come in the way people expect. And almost never does it happen that everything becomes crystal clear to them within seconds.

Instead, it is much more likely that you might notice some slight changes in the way you perceive things. The most common things people talk about centre around realizing that some of the things they previously put lots and lots of energy into might not have been quite as important as they thought. And conversely they realize that some of the things they had been neglecting might have been more important than they realized. I suspect you will have some version of this as well. But you probably won't have these realizations in the middle of treatment (well, not completely). A full processing of this will likely happen when you finish all of your treatment and have to start moving back into a structured and formal life that might look like the one you had pre-cancer.

But for now, let's focus on what happens during treatment.

During treatment

For the next weeks or months, the things that normally give you meaning and purpose might not be available to you, or at least not in the form they might have taken pre-cancer. So, the first strategy is to work out what is meaningful to you. What are the things that feel important when you do them, or what are the things that, since the cancer has come along, you haven't been able to do and have missed?

I want you to write a list of these things, then make a mark next to the ones you definitely can't do. For instance (and this is an extreme example), if you find meaning from being a competitive cyclist, but are then told you need to stay off the bike for a year, that will likely not be manageable.

But for many things on your list, I suspect that if you can't do the actual thing you might be able to change the activity slightly to make it achievable within the context of the cancer changes. For instance, if you go out for dinner each week with a large group of friends but now it feels too big and too exhausting, you might simply need to change things slightly. So perhaps you could go for coffee with a couple of friends instead. You still get the benefit of social contact and remain engaged in activities that you would normally like to do, but changing the activity will mean that you are likely to be less overwhelmed and exhausted by it. You will be able to vary most of the things you have thought about or written down, to help you continue to do those things that feel important.

If you are stuck, some examples to get you started are:
- spending time with people you like
- keeping a routine and structure for yourself and the kids
- doing puzzles
- sitting in the sunshine

- listening to the birds in the backyard
- having a tidy house
- being creative
- being able to talk about things that aren't the cancer.

The next step is to make sure these things actually get done.

Making a schedule

> Cancer is like having another full-time job. I spend all of my
> time just waiting for things to happen and I am so exhausted
> that I can't face doing anything else.
> Romesh, 44 years old

Cancer makes people busy. There are lots of appointments, time at the hospital, and time waiting for things to happen. It's usually the things that are about looking after ourselves, and the pleasurable meaningful stuff that gets dropped when there are medical things that need to be done. So I want you to make a schedule of how you are going to fit these things in. I know this sounds very rigid and probably more ordered than you would normally be, but there are so many appointments in your schedule at this time, that unless you intentionally make time to do pleasurable things they are likely to disappear. Scheduling also means that when you wake up in the morning you have a picture of what your day is going to look like — this is particularly helpful if you are feeling low in energy.

An example of scheduling might be:

7 a.m. — Wake up, have a shower, get dressed
7.30 a.m. — Breakfast while watching the news/reading the
  paper
8.30 a.m. — Walk around the block/park/house (depending on
  energy levels)

10 a.m. — Rest/watch TV

11.30 a.m. — Text friends/check social media etc.

12.30 p.m. — Lunch

1.30 p.m. — Catch up with a friend for coffee

4 p.m. — Pick up some groceries

5.30 p.m. — Dinner

7 p.m. — Watch TV/read/prepare for bed.

This may be more or less than you feel you can manage right now; it is designed to give you an idea of what to spend time on rather than being a formula. Just do what you feel is helpful for you!

It is also worth making a list of some things you can do when you are feeling low in energy that help to give you some purpose or meaning; for instance, reading a book you really enjoy, doing some knitting, or learning about something. There is a reasonable chance through the process of treatment that you will have days or times when all the things that would normally feel manageable will feel way too big. If this happens, break whatever you want to do down into smaller and smaller components until it becomes something that feels okay.

Some examples to help get you started might be:

- read a chapter of a book or read for ten minutes at a time
- crosswords
- knitting
- revisiting pleasant memories
- cleaning out one drawer/box/pile of papers
- sitting in the sunshine
- texting a friend
- taking a short walk around the neighbourhood or somewhere nice to look at
- weeding a small patch of the garden.

We will revisit the ideas around this further as we work through the book.

4.

Preparing for treatment and having a plan!

I had watched enough movies to know how bad the treatment was going to be — I couldn't possibly think of anything other than that.

Jordan, 26 years old

There is a reasonable chance that not long after you are told you have cancer, you will be given some kind of plan by your doctor or your surgeon. The plan is important in helping you move out of the sense of helplessness that sometimes comes with a diagnosis. It gives you something to do, and something to focus on.

That said, invariably whatever the plan entails will likely make you worried and anxious. That's okay. You are supposed to be worried and anxious about these things.

Before you have a plan, your brain has been given some information — information that is likely terrifying, and sitting in that space is a really difficult thing to do for too long. As we talked about earlier, this phase follows the shock of the information, and allows you to start thinking more about the future.

However, if you don't have a plan, that future can be completely overwhelming and terrifying. So although it can be scary in itself, this is when your doctor telling you that you need to have chemotherapy, surgery or radiotherapy will be comforting. The moment you are told what the plan is, you are likely to find yourself becoming focused on that, and less so on the diagnosis itself. Whenever you feel like you don't have a plan it allows your brain to spin, and likely end up at a 'worst case scenario'.

> Before they told me what I had to do, I was just floating and panicking. The doctor telling me I needed to do chemotherapy was the scariest and best thing I had ever heard.
> Mike, 57 years old

Your brain is helping you

You might also find that your mind is getting very caught up in thoughts about other plans. This might be things such as what you will do during treatment, who is going to look after the kids, how you will juggle work, etc. Again, this is your brain trying to help you out.

One of the brain's jobs is to plan and organize things for us — for instance, helping us put on matching socks in the mornings. A silly example, but a small version of thousands of decisions and actions we do every day. In the context of diagnosis and uncertainty, it makes sense that your brain might go a bit into overdrive to help you make the next part of your world as predictable as possible. So that means you are likely to start planning things in a way you have not before. This planning might help give you a sense of preparedness for what comes next. However, the trick is not to get too overwhelmed. There are lots of things to think about, and our brains can easily start to spin.

Some of the things that can be helpful here are:

- *Make a list of all the things you would normally do in a day/week.* This may feel big when you look at it initially. So, when you have your list it might be a good idea to get rid of some things straight away that don't feel important, or that you feel you don't need to worry about right now.
- *Talk to your doctor or team about what they expect you will be able to do during whatever treatment you are having.* For surgery, for instance, you might be told that you aren't able to drive for six weeks; or with chemotherapy you might be told you will be unwell for three days after treatment.
- *Think about (and maybe make a list) of the things you might need help with, or what you might be able to outsource.* For instance, if you have the resources, getting someone to mow the lawns or clean the house might take lots of pressure off you and free you up for other things.
- *Talk to the people around you and ask them to do specific things.* People will offer help but often don't know what to do. So give them a particular job, like picking up your kids from school, picking up supplies from the supermarket, etc.
- *Don't beat yourself up for asking for help.* This is a tough time, and having a plan will help you feel more prepared going forward (even if you don't need it! More about this below).

Complementary and alternative therapies

It is highly likely that at some point during your cancer experience you will consider and explore either complementary or alternative therapies. These things are very different to each other. Complementary therapies are things which are safe to have alongside your other treatments and usually have an evidence base. These might be things like oncology-specific massage, acupuncture or reflexology. These tools don't claim to have any anti-cancer effect, but are the kinds of things that might help manage symptoms like pain or nausea, and for the most part people find them pleasant to engage in.

Alternative therapies are less well accepted and have less evidence to say that they are helpful. These are things that are generally done as an alternative to traditional treatments such as chemotherapy and radiotherapy. For many promoters of these treatments, they might be unwilling or very closed to the idea of you pursuing any other treatment while you are undergoing the alternative therapy.

It can sometimes be difficult to discern the difference between complementary therapies and alternative therapies, so it is worth doing your homework from some reputable sources to understand what a particular therapy might entail and what the potential side effects might be.

If you do decide to take some herbs or supplements, it is important that you tell your doctor exactly what you are taking, because even natural things can have significant (and very dangerous) interactions with other medications. If you are not sure if something is safe, or if the claims being made about the product make you feel nervous, consult your doctor.

I was surprised. It wasn't nearly as bad as I thought.
Sam, 30 years old

How will treatment treat me?

On hearing they will need cancer treatment, most people conjure images of themselves being completely incapacitated and terribly unwell. This is based on thousands of images out there in the world and maybe the experiences of other people you know. It is important to reinforce again that every person's experience of treatment looks really different. The treatment itself might be different from person to person, even if they have the same disease. There are hundreds of types of cancer, and all of them require different treatment. So if someone in your world has leukaemia treatment, and you have breast cancer, the experiences are likely to be very different.

The other thing that happens is that as time goes on, treatment changes and side effects get managed differently. So the person who had a nasty time with treatment ten years ago is likely to have had a very different experience to what you might have now. Sometimes people are unwell with treatment; but while you might be unwell, it's likely you'll be less unwell than what you expect based on all those thousands of images.

Let's use chemotherapy as an example. If you're having three-week cycles, you might assume at the beginning that you will be unwell for the whole three weeks. What is more likely to happen is that you will be quite unwell for the first couple of days, then feel rubbish for that first week or so, but then you will hopefully start to recover. If you are well and everything is being done for you, it's likely to drive you a bit mad. In fact, having things that give you meaning and purpose are incredibly important in this space (more about this in Chapter 5).

So, if you plan for the worst-case scenario and you are actually sick and unable to get out of bed for the time you have planned for, then you are covered. And, if not, when you speak with the people who are going to help you out, tell them what you need from them; let them know you will do whatever you can, and that it's important for your recovery to do so. This will mean they understand there is some flexibility in your plans.

Here's an example: 'As you know, I am starting treatment soon. The doctors have told me that I am likely to be sick for at least a week out of the three. This means that for this week I will need some help with the kids. If I am feeling well enough, though, I would like to be able to still take them to school. Do you mind if I text you each morning to let you know if I need you to swing by on the way and pick them up?'

Generally, as long as you are able to communicate what you need, people will work out a way to support you. And if they aren't getting it, it is reasonable to be a bit blunter than perhaps you are normally.

TIPS FOR CARERS:
Supporting your person during treatment

Commencing treatment can feel like a bit of a double-edged sword for both patients and carers. Sometimes, by the time treatment comes around it will feel like you have already been completely overwhelmed by options and choices, with loads of appointments, so starting may feel like a relief. The other side of this equation, however, is the challenge of the unknown.

For you and your person, there is likely to be some anxiety about how bad the treatment might be, how well your person has planned for being unwell, and how you might juggle all the things that need to be done if your person is unwell.

The highest anxiety is likely to be during the first treatment, when things are still unknown: when waiting, for example, on the outcome of a surgery to see how recovery will look; during the first cycle of chemotherapy or immunotherapy while you wait to see if your person will be as sick as predicted; or around the commencement of radiotherapy. However, once you can get a picture of it, it is likely that you will be able to put together a plan to help make it manageable.

This uncertainty might mean it is difficult for you to anticipate how you might be able to support your person. The best way to find these things out is often to ask: 'What is it you need from me?' or 'How can I support you?'

They might initially struggle to come up with an answer, but if you leave it with them for a while they may come back to you with something. It could be really simple things. Lots of my patients speak to me about just wanting their partners to give them a hug on the lounge at night when they are watching television, or to include them in decisions about things.

5.

Chemotherapy

I remember thinking that I would spend all my time vomiting.
I was so scared. Sure, I didn't feel awesome, but I didn't
throw up once.

Nadja, 50 years old

Chemotherapy is probably one of the most well-known and often most maligned treatments for cancer. Within seconds of hearing the word most people can conjure a picture or image from a movie or television show where the main character is struck down by disease and undergoes horrendous chemotherapy. Usually, in this scenario people will have their hair fall out almost immediately, and they will be sick just as quickly, often vomiting in dramatic ways, and then just like that it is over. This, in my experience, is not like in real life, for many reasons.

First, although it makes for a good movie, uncontrolled vomiting does not make for good real life, so over the years the management of nausea and vomiting has become much better. There will be many people who are quick to tell you how horrible chemotherapy was for them or for other people in their world (and some people do have a terrible time), but this is a skewed sample. Generally, people talk much less about the things that go well for them, so if chemotherapy is manageable and okay, they aren't likely to scream it from the rooftops. Don't get me wrong, I almost never meet people who love the process of chemotherapy, but it's not about it being the best experience of your life. Chemotherapy has a job — to try to kill the cancer cells — so it just needs to be tolerable, and mostly it can be better than that.

Previously, when doctors were still trying to work out the best doses of chemotherapy for each tumour, patients might have been given big doses of drugs, which inadvertently led to more side effects. Two things have changed since then. First, the amount of drugs people get might have changed over time as doctors are able to optimize the dosage of drugs given to work on the tumours. Second, drugs called anti-emetics, which manage nausea and vomiting, were developed and are now used alongside treatment.

Effects of chemotherapy

Let's go back two steps. Chemotherapy is a treatment involving chemicals (or a combination of chemicals) that work on particular tumours. These chemicals work by attacking the cells in the body that divide rapidly (cancer cells, and some others). For each tumour type there will be a different combination of drugs given on a particular schedule, which is called a protocol. There might be some overlap between drugs and protocols for different cancers, but it is hard to generalize across protocols or cancers as each will likely have slightly different effects. Your doctor and nurses will be able to guide you about what you are having and what the most common side effects are.

I mentioned above the rapidly dividing cells. This piece is the key to side effects. Tumours are made up of cells that divide very quickly, which makes tumours grow. But our body naturally has lots of these cells — in, for instance, the lining of our mouths and digestive system, and the cells that make our hair and nails. So chemotherapy works to stop the cells in the tumour that divide very rapidly; but it also takes out some casualties: hair, stomach and other cells around the place. It is this process that causes the side effects.

The two main side effects people worry about are hair loss and nausea and vomiting. So let's chat about those first.

Hair loss

One of the biggest immediate worries most people have with chemotherapy is about hair loss. First, not all kinds of chemotherapy will cause you to lose your hair; many will, but there are some that don't cause changes at all, some that will cause hair to thin but not fall out, or it might be that your hair might change colour. Your team will be able to tell you what to expect, and give you a sense of how likely it will be that your hair will fall out.

Hair loss is horrible for most people and almost completely unimaginable for others. Often people will move between different thoughts about the process of losing their hair. One of the most difficult aspects of this can be the sense of lack of control. This would feel very different psychologically if you simply went to the barber of your own choice and asked to have your head shaved! For many people the idea of treatment itself definitely doesn't feel like a choice — they have to do everything they can to survive, which means treatment, which means side effects. Even for patients who feel completely at ease with the idea of losing their hair, when it happens it comes a shock.

It's unlikely you will have any memory of yourself without hair (unless you have intentionally shaved your head recently). The worry about losing hair is partially about fear of not knowing what you will look like, and partially about your loss of control about what is happening to you, but mostly it is around knowing what it means to not have hair. People will most likely know that you are sick.

Like many things in cancer world, the experience of losing your hair is probably not going to be as bad as you anticipate. For most people, the most intense anxiety about this is before their hair falls out, but once it happens they know there is nothing they can do and quickly come to accept it.

There are things you might be able to do to help this process along. For instance, if you have long hair, it is generally a good idea to shave it or cut it short so that you can start to make better sense of what it will mean to have less hair present.

You might also decide to get a wig so that when your hair falls out you have something to help manage when you need to be out in the world. Wigs can be very convincing, and if you get one similar to how your hair would generally look, you might be able to get away with people not necessarily knowing you have lost your hair. Around the house, though, and with the people you are close to, you might feel really comfortable not wearing anything. If you have very young children, it's a good idea to have them around when you shave your hair off — they might get very confused if there is a really big change in your appearance without them being present for it.

When your hair falls out it will likely be quite an emotional time. Often, the reality of what is happening with the cancer will hit home at this time, and you might feel quite overwhelmed. But for most people, when their hair has fallen out they work out how to make sense of it, and develop strategies to manage other people's reactions to it.

Regardless of what happens for you with respect to your body, and the changes that cancer brings, the most important thing is to allow yourself permission to grieve the loss of what you experienced from your body in the past, and work out strategies to make sense of your new relationship with your body.

Nausea and vomiting

It almost goes without saying but nausea and vomiting are very unpleasant. And, luckily for most of us, in our adult lives we don't tend to experience it very often (the most frequent experience seems to be in the context of particular overindulgence). However, when faced with chemotherapy, the fear of nausea and vomiting is one of the most frequent concerns people have. The difficulty with nausea is that it has a very good relationship with anxiety, which is where I come in.

For this to make sense, there are some important concepts to understand.

When we were evolving and being chased by lions and tigers we needed systems to keep us safe, and so our body made these for us. For instance, when we are in trouble or danger, all the blood runs from our stomachs and digestive system to our legs so they can run faster to help us escape. From time to time we still need this response, but mostly in our modern times we aren't being chased around by large jungle animals or facing big threats, so those systems might fire in a less helpful way. So, when people have chemotherapy or are unwell generally, there is a process by which that feeling of nausea and anxiety get linked together very easily.

In our brains there is a strong link between nausea, anxiety and negative things (such as being unwell). This is normally the driver for what we call 'anticipatory anxiety'. This is the anxiety that makes you feel nauseous before you've even had the chemotherapy, or sometimes before you have even made it to the hospital. The best example I have of this is a story that involves my little sister (who is now less little than she was when this story took place). When she was about three or four, she ate some fried rice with prawns in it. Coincidentally, she got gastro the next day. This took place many years go, and to this day she is unable to eat prawns. For some patients, a similar process occurs for chemotherapy, where the thought of chemotherapy (or other triggers, like the smells of the hospital) set off the anxiety response, which tells you that the whole thing is a bad idea.

We will talk about strategies to manage this above in a moment, but first — and this will sound strange — I want you to think about the worst thing that can happen from you feeling nauseous.

You might feel unwell.

It might feel difficult to do what you normally do.

You might vomit.

That's probably the worst one, right? You might vomit.

And it's unpleasant, sure. No one likes to vomit. And as an adult it rarely happens. But if that is the worst thing, then it's probably okay.

Managing worries and anxiety about chemotherapy

With anxiety, our brains go into overdrive really easily. They start worrying and constructing things that aren't really a problem. So we will revisit this concept over and over again: what is the worst thing that can happen?

When you feel yourself starting to panic about chemotherapy and potential side effects, and feel those thoughts ramping up and unravelling, just pause, and ask yourself, 'What is the worst thing that will happen?' It might be that your brain tells you myriad things — for instance, it might be that you will be too unwell to look after your kids, or that you are so sick you won't be able to get to the bathroom or make food for yourself. It can be a helpful process to work through this if it is feeling out of control in your mind.

Writing things down is likely to help give you some distance from the thoughts, so on a piece of paper I want you to write down three headings. Then think through the likely scenarios and how you might manage them. This won't get rid of the worries 100 per cent, but it is likely to help make them feel more manageable. And next time they come up, you will have a reference point to go back to.

An example might be:

What am I worried will happen?	How likely is it that it might happen?	If it did happen, how would I manage it?
That all my hair will fall out with treatment.	The doctors said there is a small chance that it might not, but it probably will.	I would hate to be caught out, so perhaps getting a wig even though I don't want to wear it would help me. I could also get some headscarves, and tell people that my hair will fall out so they won't be shocked when it happens.

Noticing three things

Now, sometimes your brain won't be satisfied with that or it might start to panic more. When we start to feel panicked or the anxious thoughts ramp up and feel really loud, one of the best things we can do is bring our focus out of our thoughts and back to the current moment (our thoughts are normally running into the future).

So, whenever your mind starts to spin with anxiety, I want you to pause and notice three things around you. These could be sounds, smells or things you can see. For example, where I am writing this, I can hear the chatter of a couple discussing what they feel like for breakfast, I can see the sun coming through the window and hitting the table, and I can smell bacon cooking on the grill. Coming back to the present, if even for a second, acts as a circuit breaker for those thoughts, and might just slow things down again. If you find yourself getting caught in those thoughts again, that's okay; just repeat the exercise and look for some more things to focus on.

Managing chemotherapy

Chemotherapy is hard to manage. Physically you will likely feel less well than normal, but also you may find you are less able to think of things to help you. Some of the strategies to manage the psychological aspects of chemotherapy can be things like:

- *Move your body.* It sounds counterintuitive, but getting out of bed and moving around, even if you just do a few laps around the house, is likely to make you feel better. Even though this will feel like a cruel irony, there is now evidence that suggests exercising when on chemotherapy helps.
- *Use your brain.* Thinking over and over again about treatment and how horrible you feel is guaranteed to make you feel worse. So having some distraction is a helpful thing. I am not talking about reading *War and Peace*, but finding something to read or something to watch that keeps your brain busy is a good plan. Often people will say that it is too hard to concentrate on reading during

treatment, but they can find audiobooks or podcasts manageable. Some use crosswords, Sudoku, etc.

- *Make a routine.* Just being on treatment will give you some routine, but making sure you have a plan for each day will help you get from one day to the next, even on the days when you feel sick. Revisit the list on page 29 where you wrote down the activities to use when you are low in energy. You might have to break these into smaller sections, but that is okay. Just do what you can manage.

- *Get dressed.* This one is particularly important if you feel unwell. It's tempting to stay in your pyjamas all day, with the covers over your head (which is okay every once in a while), but getting up, having a shower and putting on proper clothes will have a huge impact on your mood and the way you think about yourself.

- *Stay socially connected.* It's equally tempting to disconnect from people and hibernate. People do this for lots of reasons, but often it can be because they feel they don't have the energy or motivation to talk much. If this is the case, find ways of connecting with people on your terms; maybe go to a movie where you don't have to talk much, or tell a friend you can only catch up for half an hour. It's also helpful sometimes to declare a 'cancer-free zone' where they aren't able to talk about the cancer, and neither can you!

Now, I am saying all these things while feeling perfectly well. If you are feeling any less well than that, these suggestions might feel completely overwhelming. In that case, make whatever you are trying to do smaller and smaller until it feels okay. So maybe instead of going out with friends, you might send a text message, or read a magazine rather than the books you would normally manage. This cancer business is hard, so being kind to yourself and doing things, even if they feel really small, to help get you through it is the main thing.

> That first day before chemo I was distraught. How could this
> be happening to me? But then, when that first cycle was done
> I realized it wasn't nearly as bad as I had anticipated, and if I
> had to do it another four times, it would be okay.
> Linda, 45 years old

The first cycle of chemotherapy is usually the hardest psychologically, mostly because people don't know what to expect. They have thoughts and images whirring around about what it is going to be like, and will be on tenterhooks waiting to see what side effects appear. But then, after that first one, there is usually a sense of what the pattern might be, what the drugs will do, and how you will cope. Then, when these things feel more predictable it is much easier to plan and cope with it. For instance, if you know that for three days after treatment you feel rubbish, but then feel okay, you can work with that, plan some activities, work out what you want to eat (or not) and use the time when you feel well to do the things that feel the most important.

Once you find yourself in a routine with chemotherapy it will generally start to feel much easier. People normally report that after the first cycle the next couple start to feel quite manageable — they are able to plan around things, and make sense of what they need to do to make the ongoing nature of it feel okay.

If it starts to feel unmanageable

Generally, somewhere around cycle four (though this can vary from person to person) you might find it feels more unmanageable again. This is mostly due to the novelty of the treatment very much wearing off; people begin to feel that the treatment is quite unrelenting (cycle three or four is usually about halfway through treatment) and have a temporary sense that they might not be able to manage it ongoing. It's not uncommon at this time for people to report that they don't feel they can keep going with treatment, and some people may seriously consider not continuing with it. However, if you are able to reconnect with the sense of purpose and meaning we spoke about previously, and re-examine what it is you are doing to manage your sense of structure and routine, you will likely be able to get back on track.

As people go through treatment the things that might have been helping can slip away a little bit. This can happen for many reasons, including that you might be feeling better or worse physically than when you started, so the things that might help you may need to be revised and changed. Generally, once you feel back on track lots of the cycles will start to fall back into the pattern that had been working before. If they don't, and that sense that it is unrelenting is sticking around, it might be worth checking in with your team, just in case it is a sign of a bigger change in your mood (most of the time it is not, but it is worth checking in, just in case).

When chemotherapy comes to an end

The other cycle that tends to bring people undone a little bit is the penultimate one — you know, the one just before the last one. This might be the time when you realize treatment is coming to an end, or that you may have to make sense of whatever the next treatment might be; moving from chemotherapy to radiotherapy, for instance, or preparing yourself for surgery. This may also be the time in which the end starts to feel very close, but still far enough away that you have a couple of cycles ahead of you. At this time there is often a strange time parallax that happens, where time might feel as if it's slowing down and the time until the end of treatment will never come (a little bit like the time before you go on holidays). But then, conversely, the time could feel as if it is slipping away as you move quickly towards the end of treatment, and your mind might be frantically trying to make sense of what might come next (just like when you are on holidays).

It can help to reassure yourself that you will be able to manage the next part of the plan. Remember when you started chemotherapy: you were likely feeling pretty overwhelmed, and then you were able to get into the habit and routine, even if it wasn't particularly pleasant, and you didn't want to do it, but you managed it. Start to think, too, about ensuring that you maintain those strategies which have been helpful for you, and keep connecting with them. Trying to stay present and not projecting too far into the future is often really helpful — just focus on today, maybe make some plans for later in the week, but don't think too far ahead, as that's where the uncertainty lives (for more on staying present see Chapter 23).

When the last treatment rolls around you might feel quite overwhelmed by different emotions: the great pleasure of being done, but also worry about the uncertainty or plans going forward. The people around you might want to throw you a massive party or hold a big celebration, and doing this might feel okay, or it might not, and it is okay to not want to do this. Some of the people around you might not understand what it means for you to finish chemotherapy. You might feel some sadness about leaving your nurses or the other patients you have met during treatment each week. You may have been trying to ignore that worry as the days crept up, and then feel it being much more present now that treatment is really finished. Or you might not be too concerned about it at all — you might genuinely feel quite happy that it is done. Regardless, this is likely to be a time when many things feel different, and the sense of uncertainty over what happens next might be very present. It is okay to spend some time trying to make sense of this, and working with your thoughts about it. Again, as I mentioned above, if you find yourself flying too far forward into thinking about what happens next, slow down and just stay present in the moment of what is happening right now.

Chemo brain

You have probably heard the phrase 'chemo brain' used by both patients and health professionals. Simply put, it describes when people feel they are less able to manage some tasks while they are on chemo. They might feel their attention span isn't as good, or that they can't remember things quite as well. During treatment most people will experience some of these things, but most of the time when people finish treatment they will notice their cognitive skills (memory, attention, focus) start to come back to what they were before.

One of the best things to do to help manage this, even on treatment, is to use your brain, but in a way that works at that point in time. So perhaps read one chapter or read just for fifteen minutes, but don't force yourself to persevere when you become tired or unable to focus. If you are worried about how you are functioning either on chemo or when you have finished, chat with your doctor.

A note about immunotherapy

Over the past couple of years, the role of immunotherapies and other targeted therapies has become more commonplace in the management of various tumours. These may be drugs that are used by themselves or in combination with other treatments. I haven't provided much information about the side effects of these in the book for a few reasons.

First, these drugs are evolving very quickly and have different applications for different tumours, so it is hard to provide information that would be helpful. Second, anecdotally for many patients, the side effects can look quite similar to chemotherapy, but are usually tolerated quite well. Your doctor will be able to give you the specific detail about what to expect medically, but psychologically the concerns that might come up for you are likely to be pretty similar to those for chemotherapy, so the suggestions earlier in this chapter will likely be quite applicable.

TIPS FOR CARERS:
Looking after yourself during treatment

Treatment is hard work. This means that, for you as a carer, you will walk the parallel path of uncertainty and exhaustion that can come with lots of time on treatment. You will need to build resilience to help get you through. Remember how we talked earlier about putting fuel in your tank? This is one of those situations where you could easily run out of fuel if you are on auto pilot and just focusing on the person having treatment.

I would imagine one of the first things that just popped into your head might be: 'I can't do anything for myself; I don't have time.' Or perhaps 'It's not as if I am having treatment; I can't have a break while my person is going through this.' Or maybe 'I have tried that, but they always need something from me.'

I get it. It's hard to find the right balance, and I am sure you will get it wrong more than once. Almost everyone does. But what I am asking is for you to notice those thoughts that come up the second you start thinking about it. Those thoughts, particularly the ones about guilt and not looking after your person well enough, are pretty hard to feel. But they will keep turning up, so if you only listen to those thoughts this carer time is going to be really hard going.

I am not asking you to stop or get rid of the thoughts, but instead, just notice them. Knowing that these thoughts are going to turn up but then still choosing to catch up with some friends, or take up that offer of some home-cooked meals, might mean they feel much less powerful, and they might even quieten down for a bit. They will come back, but the more depleted and exhausted you feel, the stronger such thoughts will feel.

It's simple to find many examples of things that will likely help when you are feeling good. But if you are feeling exhausted it might be tough to come up with even a few things to help you feel better. If you are struggling with this, perhaps it might be worth sitting down and coming up with a list. These things could range from really small (like reading a paragraph of a book), through to bigger (going to the gym for an hour) or really big (getting away for a whole day or weekend). But if you manage to do a couple of these things every day it will help protect you a bit from the challenges of trying to keep the tank full when there is a really big hole draining the fuel out!

6.

Radiotherapy

I know that it is ridiculous, but every time I think about
radiotherapy I picture a super villain attacking me with
radioactive waste. I don't think that the imagery is helping me.
Amaya, 29 years old

The imagery around radiotherapy can be enough to make people baulk at
it. And they do. People often have the idea that something radioactive is
going to happen, which makes it sound overwhelming and terrifying. The
reality is, though, that the process of radiotherapy is often just like having
an X-ray or a CT scan. The treatment itself is painless while you are having
it and the side effects occur towards the end of treatment, rather than the
whole way through.

Simply put, radiotherapy is the process of using targeted X-rays to
shrink tumours. Just like chemotherapy, lots of the horror stories come
from a time in history when the thoughts were that the more treatment
the better, and over time the techniques as well as approaches to delivering
radiotherapy have improved significantly, with people needing smaller and

smaller areas treated, meaning less healthy tissue is involved (read: fewer side effects).

There are some general side effects for radiotherapy, mostly involving skin irritation at the site of treatment and fatigue. Both tend to arrive towards the end of treatment, continue for a couple of weeks afterwards, then start to improve. The management of skin irritation is quite standard and all patients will be given creams and recommendations. The fatigue, somewhat like chemotherapy fatigue, is managed mostly by listening to your body and balancing the need to rest with the need to move and have some purpose. Generally, people find that doing things and keeping their bodies moving is better than not!

However, depending on the site of treatment, you may experience more specific side effects or difficulties. For instance, if your tumour is in your pelvis and you have radiotherapy to your abdomen, you might experience difficulties with your bowels during treatment. Similarly, if you are having treatment to your neck, you might have a sore throat and difficulties in swallowing. If you are likely to have specific side effects your doctor will explain these in full before you commence treatment.

Psychological difficulties during radiotherapy

There are some common difficulties people have during radiotherapy which I will outline below along with some simple strategies to try to manage them.

Claustrophobia

For some cancers, usually ones in the head and neck, you might be required to wear a radiotherapy mask which is made to fit your face, to ensure that when treatment is being delivered you don't move. There may also be some other situations when people might find themselves feeling confined and feeling overwhelmed, for instance if you are told that you have to hold still and not move.

For many people, the first couple of times they wear the mask or have treatment might feel difficult, but then as time goes on, they feel like they can manage okay. However, if you are feeling that you can't manage or that the feelings are getting worse, it is always important to tell your treatment team, as they have some things that will likely help (this is a very common problem). Having something else to think about or be distracted by is simple yet works really well. Ask the team to play you some music to tune into while you are being treated, then try to focus on just one instrument (drums work well because they are often a bit unpredictable and you have to really pay attention) or think of things you can do with your brain, such as trying to replay the start of your favourite movie, or a scene from a television show you really like, list off the ingredients and steps in a recipe you make a lot, or think of a trip you would like to take. It doesn't really matter what you think about, as long as it is sticky enough to distract you. You might find your mind will wander back to the room and the mask or the feelings of being trapped; that's okay, just shift them back again to what you would like to think about. There will always be some strategies to help you manage this, so if you are struggling with it, ask!

The unrelenting nature of treatment

Most radiotherapy treatment courses will run over at least five to six weeks. Every weekday. Generally, this happens at the same time each day with a break on the weekends. For most people this takes some organizing and planning, and is usually reasonably disruptive.

The biggest difficulty people have in managing radiotherapy is usually related to tolerating its ongoing nature. But there are some pluses to this. Remember how in the chemotherapy section we spoke about the importance of routine and structure? Well, radiotherapy provides that structure, which for many people is a bit of a relief coming out of a much less structured treatment or when recovering from surgery. However, if this is the only structure in your day, or you perceive that the radiotherapy is getting in the way of you being able to do other things, like going back to work, then your relationship to radiotherapy is likely to be more problematic. As we spoke about earlier, one of the ways of managing any of these treatments is having some structure and purpose; if you feel you are not managing the process well, it is worth asking yourself the question, 'What is driving the problem?' Is it around your general frustration and being 'over' everything, or is it related to specific aspects? Is it about your difficulties in managing the travel to and from the centre, or is your life revolving around the treatment? Each of these concerns will require a very different intervention and process. We will cover most of these concerns as we work our way through the book.

7.

Surgery

I knew that when I woke up my leg would be missing — but I didn't really understand what it would mean. Not until I was sitting there just looking at the space where it used to be.
Liyang, 45 years old

Surgery is one of the big variables in the cancer space. For some, their experience of surgery might feel so small that it barely registers, but for others it might be the thing that feels the most significant in this whole cancer experience.

Surgery might be one of the first things that happens for you — and for lots of people there will be at least a small surgical procedure to determine the nature of your cancer (such as a biopsy or lymph node removal). For others, though, there can be many other treatments before surgery comes into the picture. The size and detail of surgeries can look really different, even between people who have similar cancers, and it is worth speaking with your surgical team about what exactly you can expect or what the potential difficulties might be. This isn't about scaring you; this is about setting realistic expectations. For instance, lots of my patients cope much better if they know up front they are going to be in hospital for three weeks rather than going in under the assumption they will be in for a week, and then realizing this won't be the case. I can guarantee you that the person who has planned for a three-week admission and has thought about what they will do to manage this, can usually cope much better than someone who thinks they will be in for a week and ends up being in for three! Also, asking your surgeon to be realistic with you about what is likely to happen after the surgery will help you prepare. So if you are not going to be able to eat for a couple of days, or if you are going to wake up in the ICU or with lots of drains, it can make a huge difference in how you make sense of this if you have some preparation around it.

What's different about surgery?

Psychologically there are some things which make surgery different than other treatments.

You will be put to sleep

This is a weird concept for us to get our heads around, particularly if you haven't had the experience before. It's very common for people to be anxious about what might occur if something happens and they don't wake up. It is also generally difficult for people to make sense of how to be absent, and missing sometimes long periods of time.

In many ways the experience of going for surgery and being absent feels difficult and hard to reconcile, and it makes sense that people might feel anxious and overwhelmed by this process. For the most part, there is nothing you can specifically do to override this, but for lots of my patients it helps a little to feel that practical things have been arranged. These might be things such as having some of those difficult conversations about what you might like to happen if something did happen to you, writing a will or telling people things that feel important to you; this might help you feel reassured, just in case anything was to happen. This is a little bit like an insurance policy: hopefully you don't need it, but having it in place will help you feel reassured that there is a plan if the worst was to happen.

You are scared of what will happen when you wake up

People are often pretty quick to dispense advice about how difficult things can be post-surgery. It wouldn't surprise me if you someone tells you some kind of post-surgery horror story that will invariably freak you out. You yourself might have had a difficult time with a procedure or surgery in the past, which could make you feel much more worried.

Of course, there is always a chance things won't go as planned, but for the most part this is a small chance. Surgeons (and doctors in general, for that matter) do a very good job at explaining the risks of a procedure, so it is likely that when you consent for your surgery, you will have a good idea of what those risks are. That said, any risk might feel very big and significant. For you, it is likely the first time you've had this particular surgery, but your surgeon has probably done hundreds if not thousands of surgeries that look exactly like yours. Ask them what you should expect when you wake up — and get them to be explicit. If they say you will wake up with a tube in, get them to tell you why, how long it's likely to be there for after you wake up, and what the plan is for getting it out. You are likely to worry about these things anyway, so having a plan will help you manage. This is also true in the days and weeks after your initial recovery — if you know that it is going to be six weeks before you can get back to doing what you normally do, make a plan of not only how you will manage the time in hospital but in the weeks after. This might include storing up a favourite television show to watch, or revisiting some books you really like. If you don't have a plan, lying around and waiting for the time to pass will feel very torturous and overwhelming.

You are scared of pain

There is a likelihood that if you have had surgery there may be some pain associated when you wake up and the anaesthetic has worn off. Usually, when you wake up there will be many drugs to help you manage the pain, and the nurses in particular are likely to ask you many times a day whether you have pain. Most people can recognize pain that is intense, but might not view discomfort or inability to settle as pain; these can both be a sign of the pain itself, or a sign that the pain medications are wearing off. So being alert to your early signs that the pain medication might be wearing off is a good way of taking action and staying on top of the pain, rather than the other way around.

Lots of people worry about taking pain medications in case they get addicted, but in an acute cancer setting this almost never happens (and if it did your team would work out a plan to manage it!). It is much better that you have your pain well controlled to allow you to be able to get out of bed, move around, shower, etc., which is ultimately what will help you get home.

There might be some situations where you may have pain; for instance, if you have been in bed for some time and then have to get up and move around you might have some expected pain. But even then, there is usually a plan to help you manage. Generally, after you have had surgery your pain management will be well looked after. As above, though, if you are worried about it, ask your surgeon and their team to go through what to expect and then have a plan.

You are worried your body won't look the same

As we talked about before, there are lots of different types of surgeries and as a result there will be lots of different types of changes you will have in your body. Some people will have almost no change. For instance, a small biopsy may leave almost no physical changes, while others will experience significant changes such as the loss of a limb or breast, a loss of part of an organ, a big scar or a stoma. The way you manage these things looks different from person to person — many of my patients who have had amputations, for instance, are able to adjust easily, while others with seemingly smaller residual impacts have found it more difficult.

Often, the way you frame the loss (or gain) can help you make sense of it. If, for example, you are confident that by having a particular surgery you remove any future chance of the cancer returning, it may feel quite okay to then manage the changes. However you make sense of it, it is important to recognize the loss as just that: a loss. If you had an accident and woke up suddenly without something you wouldn't expect to be okay with it straight away — this process is the same. With any grief it takes time to make sense of the changes and what it means for you going forward. If you are struggling with this, it is probably worth looking at Chapter 20 about body image.

Summary of Part 1
On treatment

There is no doubt that being diagnosed and starting treatment can be huge and overwhelming. Hopefully, though, by reading through the chapters in Part 1 you have been reassured that lots of the things that are happening for you emotionally are pretty expected. Remember, if you haven't had something like this happen before it can take your brain a bit of time to make sense of it.

Here are some key things to remember.

Understand that you will have worry and anxiety

Many people will be familiar with anxiety, but lots of others might never have experienced it before. But more often than not, when cancer comes along people feel more anxious than they have in the past — worrying about the future, about treatment, etc. The most important thing is not trying to get rid of the anxiety (that will take lots of energy and probably won't get you anywhere), but instead allowing it to be present and being kind to yourself.

Come up with a plan

When you know what the plan is, you are going to feel more settled and you will have something to work towards. If you aren't able to achieve this in the context of treatment (as it sometimes takes the teams a little while to work out the best way of managing things) then you can make your own plan. Start small: what do you need to do in the next hour, the next day and maybe even the next week? Writing this down can help make things feel more manageable.

Work out what you want people to know

Having lots of support can be as overwhelming as having none. It can be helpful to work out what you want to communicate to the people in your world, but also think about what you need them to do. If you can direct them in how best to support you, it will mean they will feel like they are being helpful, but also that you will get the support you need.

Expect that you will go up and down

Some days this will all feel completely manageable; other days you will want to hide in your bed away from the world. As long as that feeling doesn't go on for too long, it's okay. This is a tough thing to deal with, so we expect there will be some up and down.

Part 2

Off treatment

Shaun's life looked pretty different from when he didn't have cancer to when he did.

Before his cancer he was at university, and he was struggling with it. He was studying accounting but he hated it. He kept going, though, because he wasn't sure what else to do. But when the cancer came, and he wasn't able to study any more, the last thing he wanted to do was to go and sit in a dark lecture theatre listening to an old guy talk about accounting theory.

Shaun didn't mind treatment too much; it was just that he felt sick so much of the time. But he made lots of jokes with his friends that he was smashing out more binge watching than anyone else he knew. He was able to watch all the shows he had ever even thought about watching, and at the beginning he thought he would never get bored of it. It was nice to just not need to do anything other than be sick — for a while. Then the boredom crept in, just before his surgery where he had his knee replaced, and then he was on crutches for what felt like months.

Shaun knew that his mates didn't really know what to talk about with him. He looked different, and felt different, and they couldn't do the things they had done before. Before the cancer, they spent most of their weekends together playing rugby then going to the pub. It wasn't that he wasn't allowed to drink — his doctor said that he could — but he didn't really want to. He would see pictures of everyone on social media out doing things, and he would feel the anger start to arrive. It was strange; he didn't want to be doing some of the things he got angry about, but it was almost as if he didn't want other people to be doing them, either. Shaun's life had stopped, and he knew that it would restart, but in the meantime he couldn't believe that the people around him were just continuing on as if nothing had changed. Everything had changed: the way he walked, the way he thought about things, what he wanted to do with his life.

When treatment finished, Shaun couldn't imagine what it would be like to go back to everything, just as if nothing had happened. So he didn't really. He sat around the house, kept watching TV, did some physiotherapy occasionally, and spoke with his mates via text. He went out for a mate's birthday, and met a girl he liked, but freaked out at the idea that she would be interested in him. Could he tell her about the cancer; should he tell her about it? If she was into him, how would he explain the scars and weird things that went on in his body after treatment? How could he explain that he couldn't really run or do lots of other things pretty normal for a young person, like even walking on soft sand?

Shaun started questioning what it meant for him to go forward from the end of treatment — he never realized treatment would actually be the easy part in all of this. He was shocked by how much he found himself worrying about the future, and whether the cancer would come back. When it happened the first time he was so surprised by it; he hadn't really thought about it at all. But knowing there was a chance it could come back was much harder to get out of his head. Every time he felt something strange in his body he was sure it was a sign the cancer had returned. He was going to the GP several times a week, and each time he waited for the doctor to tell him the cancer was back and there was nothing they could do. He didn't want to do anything just in case it did come back, because what's the point of making plans that won't end up happening?

Shaun decided he had to find another way of thinking about the cancer, because it was taking over his life. He spent lots of time thinking about what he wanted his life to look like if he was going to die. The first couple of times that he thought about this it freaked him out, and he was terrified. But then, he found that thinking about life in this way allowed him to be less fearful of it. He was able to think about what felt important, and over time he was able to understand that he couldn't fight against the cancer — it would do whatever it wanted to do. But he knew that if it came back, he would work out a way to manage it, just like he had the first time around. So, instead he decided it was more important to find some things that felt helpful and important in his life.

8.

Finishing treatment

I thought that the second I was be done I'd be dancing in the street. Instead, I found myself with this emptiness and loss that I couldn't explain or anticipate.

Lorraine, 60 years old

Logically, it makes sense that people would be happy or excited about treatment ending — particularly for those where it has been especially hard going or long term. But what can come along for people at the end of treatment might feel like quite a surprise.

For many people, there is an expectation that the end of treatment will herald the end of their suffering and difficulties with cancer, and will mean that the elusive normality they have been craving will be able to return. However, in reality, the psychological processes around finishing cancer treatment look a little different. Many people notice more worries and thoughts about finishing as they near the last treatment/s, and will start to anticipate what things will look like when treatment is done. They may feel more anxious, and experience a sinking feeling when the people around them talk about having a party to celebrate the end of treatment, or talking about the future. This feeling is also likely to be present in that last treatment, where saying goodbye to the nurses and radiation therapists who have given you all of your treatment will feel overwhelming, and you may feel a sense of loss at knowing you are finished.

Following the end of treatment, some people experience a temporary euphoria that might last for a couple of days. But more commonly in the days or week after finishing treatment, most find themselves feeling quite lost and overwhelmed by not being quite sure how to make sense of all of this.

As with most big experiences that happen in life, it rarely makes sense to try to process the emotions around it at the same time that you are trying to make decisions and prepare for whatever is to come. This is especially true if you became very unwell very quickly and had to make decisions equally fast. But, just like the equation about energy conservation that you would have learned in high school (you remember the one: where there is energy of some description that just gets shifted from one object to another — it doesn't disappear), the emotion from that time is conserved, and it will appear somewhere else. Finishing treatment is often the sign to your brain that the physical piece is done, and now it's time for the emotional bit to kick in.

Now, I appreciate that the idea of having to manage the emotion might sound completely overwhelming when you are already so exhausted, but let's talk about how to manage at least some of it.

Give yourself time

On that last day of treatment I was excited, I couldn't wait to get back to my old life. But then in the days afterward I struggled to remember what my old life was exactly, and I definitely wasn't sure about how to find my way back to it.
Jess, 37 years old

When people finish treatment, there is often a sense of pressure 'to get back to normal' but there is wisdom in giving yourself time to try to make some sense of everything that has just happened. And just like that summer after school finishes and real life starts, you aren't likely to get the time to do it after you go back to work or when people around you have seen that you have recovered. It's an important time to allow yourself the space to process everything that has happened. When I say process, I don't mean that you will necessarily get to a space where it all makes sense, but perhaps instead it is about allowing yourself the time to know that you need to think about it, rather than just running quickly to the next thing.

Following are three steps that can help you start to make sense of your experience.

Anticipate mixed emotions

One of the first steps in managing this is anticipating that you will have emotions around finishing treatment. These could look like sadness or grief or fear, or many others. But you should anticipate that it is pretty likely these things will come up. They do for almost everyone. Some people are convinced that it won't happen to them, and so when it does they find themselves floored and overwhelmed. But, if you assume that at least in some way this is likely to be problematic for you, it enables you to name it and work with it. If you know that these emotions are likely to be present, you can work to come up with some strategies to help manage them.

A way of doing this can be to actually have that conversation with your brain. When thoughts about the future and feelings of overwhelm start to come up, just mention to yourself that this is a normal part of the process post-treatment, and allow yourself to recognize that this time is important.

Stay present

As a natural part of all this you might find that your mind shifts between thinking about the past (including everything that has just happened) and the future, where everything might feel much less certain. Connecting with the sense of being present can anchor you back into the now. Getting present can be very simple: it might be noticing a sound you hear in the room, or tuning in to your breathing. It might be as simple as telling yourself that right here, right now in this moment, you are okay. This will hopefully, even in a temporary way, help you be more able to manage the thoughts that are flying around.

Give yourself a break

Once you have allowed these worries to be around, and have some strategies to help you stay present, the third step is to give yourself a break from it.

Thinking about this stuff all the time can be exhausting, especially when you are likely to already be feeling exhausted. So it's important to find some ways to give yourself a break from thinking about it. That said, these ways need to feel valuable and important, not just serve as a distraction from the discomfort of thinking about things. Think about the things you value, and do things that are in accordance with those. It's not about getting rid of the thoughts or stopping yourself thinking about the past or the future, and it's definitely not about getting you over it so you can 'get back to normal'. It's just about giving you some nourishment. So find some nice things that make you feel good, and put some of those in your day (even if it feels really indulgent).

> I felt like the thoughts about the cancer returning would go —
> but they still appear even now, a long time after treatment is
> done. They are the worst in the days before I see my doctor.
> Each time I think they won't show up, but there they are in
> my mind in the days before I get my scan results.
> Chetna, 45 years old

Acceptance

Like many a bad Hollywood quote I am going to tell you that the first step is acceptance. And when I say acceptance, I don't mean being unquestionably happy and joyful at the presence of this worry and anxiety in your world. Instead, I want you to accept its presence. We have talked about this before and we will talk about it again and again in the context of this kind of anxiety.

I have met people who want so badly for these thoughts and anxieties to be gone, but it seems that the more they fight with them, the bigger and more difficult they become. But if you know that this anxiety about the cancer returning is what's meant to happen, and you can make room for it to be there, then that is much more manageable than fighting against it. When it arrives, perhaps it is about welcoming it like an old friend dropping in for a cup of tea: 'Ah, anxiety, I have been waiting for you to arrive.'

I appreciate that allowing it to be there might be pretty challenging, but I like to think of it like this. I want you to picture a balloon, maybe a red one, on a string on your wrist. Then, imagine you are walking down a street and the wind is blowing the balloon around behind you. But then the wind changes, and sometimes the balloon just hits you in the face, just for a second before it changes direction again and you carry on.

The worry or anxiety about this stuff is the balloon, and sometimes it will hit you in the face. At the moment, if you have just finished treatment it's much more likely to hit you in the face than it will be in a little while; and a while after that it might only hit you occasionally. But the balloon will always be there.

The important part of this story is that even though getting hit with the balloon is unpleasant, it doesn't hurt you, and it is okay.

The anxiety is the same. It's not going to hurt you, it's just your brain trying to help you, and as time goes on you will get better at knowing which way the wind is blowing.

TIPS FOR CARERS:
Finishing treatment

Great! Treatment is over, so everything can go back to normal now. Right? Well, not exactly. In fact, this might be the time for both you and your person when the enormity of what has just happened will feel even bigger. While on treatment there are lots of distractions and things to keep you busy; whereas when treatment stops your brain actually has time to catch up with what has happened and process some of the emotions behind it.

You might find yourself feeling more fearful and overwhelmed now that you don't feel as if 'anything is being done' to keep the cancer at bay.

You might find yourself thinking more about the future and questioning what you feel is important. It may be that you actually start to deliberate over whether you are doing the right things with work, friends, or even your relationship.

You might worry about the cancer coming back in a way you haven't thought about before (even if you have been reassured that it isn't likely to come back). Or you might not experience any of these things, and it could feel like it is all done and dusted. Regardless, it might be that the person you have been caring for all this time might have similar or very different feelings.

If you and your person are on different pages about this, it is likely to cause friction. The best way to manage this is to communicate what is happening for you and find out what is happening for them. Often people will work hard to protect each other, and unless you have an honest conversation about it, it might be that no one is saying what is really happening for them, leaving the other person in the dark. I am relatively sure that if you are feeling fearful about the cancer returning you will be pretty hesitant to bring that up with your person. You might be worried about them getting distressed or upset, or perhaps because they are always positive you might think they haven't thought about it at all.

Guess what? They have thought about it. And if you are worried, there is a good chance that they are worried too. If you are able to name it and talk about it, then you can do something about it. The elephant is in the room, but you can see it and talk about it, maybe even talk to it! This is a much better option than both carrying it around and not knowing how to manage it, even if that first conversation feels really hard.

9.

What if it comes back?

When an ache happened in the past it was probably just an ache, something that happened when you moved furniture about, or when you did a spectacular move that you wouldn't normally bust out on the dance floor. But an ache isn't just an ache anymore is it? Now, it might be all of the above things, or it might be something much more sinister, perhaps a signal that the cancer has returned?

Tam, 43 years old

There are very few, if any, people I have encountered who do not think about their cancer returning. They might not think about it constantly, or in a conscious way; but most people will, at the end of their treatment, find themselves thinking or worrying about what might happen if the cancer was to come back.

Before I go on, I feel it is important to point out that there is absolutely no evidence that thinking about the cancer coming back is related in any way to the cancer actually coming back. The cancer will do what the cancer will do, and you thinking about it can't change that (despite what you might have heard). In addition to this, lots of people become overwhelmed with the idea that being stressed will make their cancer return. As far as I am aware, there have been no studies that have shown a direct link between stress and cancer recurrence. That said, living a life that is less stressful isn't a bad thing to do, but it's generally not helpful to beat yourself up if you experience stress. Stress is a normal and expected part of life.

Many people will fight and fight and fight with their brain to not have thoughts about it coming back, and then find that those thoughts keep coming up anyway. Let's take a step back and think about what the mechanism is for our brains. In the not-too-distant past you probably found yourself in a situation that resulted in you not being able to trust your body in the way you would have before. Previously, there might have been things that happened which you wouldn't have thought about twice, even if you were quite tuned in to your body. But now, it is likely you will analyze any ache or pain with a level of scrutiny you hadn't before. You are on high alert because you have been caught out before, and you don't want it to happen again.

In psychology land we call this hypervigilance, or being very aware of the threat of danger in the world. This translates into being more anxious around anything that is likely to be a threat. This is a mechanism that occurs when there have been circumstances where someone has either had something bad happen or where there was potential for something bad to happen.

Think about the last time you crossed the road. If a car came from nowhere and almost hit you, giving you a pretty decent scare, I'm willing to bet that the next time you go to cross the road you'll feel more anxious and apprehensive about stepping out.

So, your brain is trying to help you out. It is trying to think of every scenario to help protect you from being caught unawares again. That means you are now thinking and being much more present to the threat of something bad happening. And in the context of this it will likely mean you are going to be thinking more and more about the future and what would happen if the cancer did return.

Sometimes these thoughts can be quite dark, and you might project into a future where you think about the worst-case scenario for you. For your brain it makes sense that thinking into this future might help you manage the situation if the cancer did return. It is likely to go into overdrive and interpret information from lots of different sources as evidence that your cancer has returned or might return.

Cancer everywhere

> And all of a sudden everywhere people not only had cancer, but the television was only covering cases where their cancer had come back and they were going to die.
> Michelle, 55 years old

When you have cancer it's a little like when you buy a new car. All of a sudden, you will notice the same car everywhere, even though you had never noticed it before. The television and newspapers have always been filled with cancer stories, it's just that now they feel more connected to you than they have been before. When you feel anxious or overwhelmed about the cancer coming back, you may be more tuned in to any of these stories that appear, and you might interpret these situations as evidence that the same will happen to you.

I am going to say some controversial things now, some of which might be hard to read, but stick with me.

The root of the fear of the cancer coming back is largely about you being fearful of dying. There are some other parts to it (like being fearful of having treatment again, or worrying about how you might cope next time around), but for the most part the anxiety is very much about what would happen if it came back and you were to die.

I imagine the paragraph above was pretty difficult to read. Perhaps you've already identified this as the driver for your anxiety but have been too scared to allow it to be present. Or you might have been fighting against it and not allowing the thoughts to be present at all. Interestingly, what often happens is that in allowing those thoughts to be present you might find they become less overwhelming and scary. Sometimes naming the thing that you fear most allows you to be present to it in a way that you might not be able to normally.

Will it feel comfortable or okay? Probably not. Instead, I suspect it will be the opposite, and those first few times you start to explore it, it might feel completely overwhelming. But over time, it's likely that making some room for making sense of it will allow it to feel more manageable. Not okay, or pleasant, but manageable.

Some more reassurance

There are some other factors that might help reassure you and manage this fear.

First, even if you haven't been told about it, it's likely that your doctors will have a plan for if your cancer returned. And if they didn't have a plan they would communicate this to you. In some ways it doesn't matter what the plan is; the important thing is that the plan exists. Often just knowing this is in itself enough to allay some of the anxiety.

The other factor is that if your cancer were to return, you would likely manage it in the same way you did the first time around. Think back to six months before your diagnosis — if someone had told you that you were going to have cancer, you would not have been able to conceptualize how you would manage it, and in all likelihood would convince yourself that you wouldn't be able to manage it at all. But like many things in life, when situations present themselves you go into action mode and work out how you will get through it.

If your cancer comes back, it will be exactly the same: you will get on and manage it however you need to.

10.

Finding your purpose and meaning:
part 2

I just kept waiting to wake up and for everything to make
perfect sense about what I wanted my future to be. It just
never happened for me.
Amanda, 52 years old

Finishing treatment can present a series of challenges. Some of these are
physical, but many more revolve around the psychological challenges of
what it means to have had such a big thing happen to you, and then to reconcile what happens next.

There is often also an aspect of trying to work out what all of this actually means. The process of treatment and the initial part of being unwell is
largely about survival. Our brains and bodies are able to engage with strategies that help make the situation tolerable — doing whatever you can just

to make it through a pretty unpleasant time. At those moments, it is largely unhelpful for you to be connected to any emotional processing of what is happening to you, or around what might happen next. Obviously, in the midst of all of it you will still have emotional responses, but they aren't likely to involve thinking deeply about the purpose or meaning of this going forward. Instead our brain is able to focus much more on the right now.

It is not uncommon in the midst of treatment for people to have some thoughts, or at times fantasies, about the future, and what that future might look like. But it is often not until treatment is finished that the questions around how to put these things into place in a real way become a possibility.

A change in priorities

As I mentioned earlier, it's a misunderstanding that people experience an incredible epiphany in the wake of their cancer experience or diagnosis. Very occasionally, I have met people who do truly have significant changes in the way they view the world and all the things they have been doing. Such people undergo a complete re-evaluation and exploration around priorities, and make big decisions (like leaving a partner or moving overseas) but this is very much the exception. Rarely, it seems, does having cancer provide people with clarity or all the answers they may have been seeking or awaiting. Much more often, people experience a slight change in priorities, or a movement towards or away from something they had been doing.

If, for example, you have been working a lot prior to the diagnosis, you might decide to change your working patterns to allow more time with your family or friends. Conversely, it might be that prior to becoming unwell you felt unsatisfied or bored with your life and might look to develop new interests or pursuits that feel meaningful or important for you.

Of course, it is perfectly reasonable in the context of having had a life-threatening experience that you might focus on things that feel most important and working out ways to manage these. Most people report that very early after the completion of treatment their awareness of the fragility of life and the need to make the most of every moment is the strongest, but then this fades gradually as they become immersed back into their previous habits. There can be an incredible pressure that comes from feeling you have to make the most of everything, and ensure that every experience feels inherently meaningful. Of course, some things will feel meaningful, and being present to them is an incredibly important thing; however, there will be just as many things in your life that will need to be done out of necessity, and might not feel quite as meaningful (doing chores around the house, for instance). Putting pressure on yourself to experience everything at this level of intensity can be very exhausting.

For many people, the idea of losing the connection to this sense of fragility can be terrifying. Generally, people worry that if they forget the experience of the cancer and how it felt, they will go back to living their lives in the same way as previously and they're scared that all the lessons learnt will quickly be lost. Although many people report that their feelings around this change somewhat over time, they are unlikely to forget it and instead make some changes to their lives that enable them to sustain the things they noted to be the most important as they worked their way through their cancer and treatment.

What feels important for you?

So, one of the first questions to ask yourself following the completion of the treatment is, what feels important for you right now? What have you come to realize that you value in a different way than perhaps you did before? What do you want to hold onto as a result of your cancer experience? Depending on how you like to think about things, it might even be worth sitting down with a piece of paper and a pen (it works better to do this stuff analogue than on a device) and list all the things that feel important to you right now. Then when you have a list, think about the ways you can act to make sure these things happen — having a thought about something feeling important and then not being able to access that is likely to make you feel quite unsatisfied.

Perhaps, for example, you identify that you really value having good relationships, as you feel that through the cancer the people around you took on more importance than they had previously when you were distracted by other things. In this case, you'd think through the situations in which you can build and nurture your relationships. So you might decide you'll organize a family dinner each week with your siblings, or set aside an hour each weekend to meet a friend in the park with your kids.

This technique will work with most values or ideas around things that are important to you. If the value is something that feels really nebulous for you, perhaps break that down a little into smaller, more manageable chunks. For instance, if you have decided that following your cancer you feel you need to prioritize the financial security of your family, it may seem very overwhelming in that state. However, it could be more easy to manage if you think separately about insurance, putting some money away for the future, paying off the house, etc., and come up with a separate strategy for each of these pieces.

Other changes after treatment

As with anything we have talked about in the context of the transition into the future following treatment, it might be that the people around you don't understand your reasons for wanting to change your priorities. We as humans build friendships and relationships, and then over time they are likely to fall into a pattern of behaviour where each person will bring certain aspects of themselves into the way you interact together. So, if this suddenly changes, it might be that there are some changes within the relationship itself. Imagine (and this is a simple example) you and a friend have always gone out to the pub on a Sunday afternoon for a couple of drinks and a pretty hefty chicken schnitzel. Following your cancer you feel that changing your diet and lifestyle habits is much more important to you but your friend hasn't changed; there is likely to be some tension around how you spend your time together. There might be some simple solutions: for instance, you might be happy to keep going to the pub but drink water and have a salad; or it might be that when you suggest changing the habit to go for a walk somewhere nice instead they happily go along. But there is a chance they might not want to change the routine, or not understand why you want to make these changes, which is likely to be quite frustrating and put a strain on the relationship. If this is the case, you might find yourself evaluating the relationship itself, and may even make a decision to not spend as much time with the person.

It is worth mentioning that many of the people I see notice a significant change in the way they perceive the world following treatment, and also in the way they perceive other people's worlds or concerns. Generally, going through treatment can be one of the most difficult things that life will have thrown at you; in some ways this provides an excellent reference point to put things into perspective and work out how you can make meaning in your life by not getting caught up in things that don't feel quite as important as they may have in the past. However, it isn't likely that other people will have had their perspective changed in this way, so they will continue to experience the world in the same way, with a focus on things that perhaps you now feel are quite unimportant and insignificant. It isn't out of the realm of possibility that we have had friends who are caught up in something that is going on for them which we don't think is very important, and we get very frustrated about them not being able to move on. For many people post-treatment this feeling can be amplified and they may find many of their social interactions quite challenging. I like to think of this as similar to being really proficient at something, say speaking French. If you know the language and its nuances well, it's easy for you to understand a person who has done a couple of lessons and is testing out their new learning on you. But it doesn't work in reverse: just because you understand them, doesn't mean they will understand you, because they don't have the same level of skill. In this situation you are the person who has the insight about what feels important and meaningful, and you are trying to communicate this to people who don't understand the language. It isn't any failing on their part; it's just that they haven't had the experience you have had to make this kind of distinction in the world. So, I encourage you to just notice your experience of frustration and sense of disconnect, and then be present to them in the same way the advanced language teacher helps a less experienced student learn.

Making sense of the changes and moving forward

Over time you might find that some of the things that feel most important at the completion of treatment feel much less important as you get back into more of a routine or a structure. Or you might be uncertain about what to do with some things right now, so you let them wander around in your mind for a little while before you work out how to bring them into action. Regardless, it is worth noticing these things and allowing them to be part of your world. Making sense of the things that have changed as a result of your cancer experience is an important part of processing everything that has happened, as is making sense of what is to come next. Allow yourself the time and space you need, and try not to be too worried about rushing into the next part just yet.

> After my world was turned upside down I was able to get everything back to 'normal', but the way I felt has never quite gone back to how I was before the cancer — maybe it never will. And now, I think maybe that isn't a bad thing.
> Paola, 58 years old

Unfortunately, sometimes your world might change in a way that feels irreparable once you finish treatment. This could be due to physical or emotional changes, or it may be that you make a choice to make changes (such as retiring early or changing jobs). Either way, you are likely to feel that you have some significant work to do around thinking about how you will find meaning and purpose going forward.

If you feel unsure about what is important to you it might be helpful to reconnect with your values. What are the things that, despite everything, still feel important? This might be connections with people, feeling a sense of purpose, how you spend your time or how you find meaning. I imagine your head might be spinning a bit reading that last sentence, but the process itself can be much easier to connect with than you might think. Think about those moments when things weren't feeling so good — what were the things that you craved or wanted to connect to? Some patients find they can clearly think of the things that felt really important, such as spending time with family, or having things to do that kept them feeling occupied, or feeling like they had some purpose (even if it felt small). Thinking about your values might be a helpful way to direct what you want to do with your time.

TIPS FOR CARERS:
At the end of treatment

Many patients return to their pre-cancer 'normal', like being back at work, managing all the balls they were juggling before, and even exercising and socializing. This doesn't mean that the struggle of making sense of the cancer has gone — in fact, this might be the time when they need more emotional support from you. This might be the time where asking the question of what your person needs from you will be one of the most helpful things you can do.

Conversely, though, it might be a helpful question to ask yourself. Just as it has been a really difficult time for the patient, it has also been a tough time for you as a carer. What do you need to help nourish and support you emotionally? Are there things you and your person can do together that will help both of you through this really difficult time? Is it that you need to have some time where you talk about the cancer and what has changed for you since it appeared? Or perhaps you don't want to talk about it at all. Are there things that you have stopped doing because of the cancer or your role as a carer that you can restart to help you feel more settled?

It is common for people to notice a slight shift or change in their values following big life events. This might include you revisiting or reconsidering some of the things you previously thought were really important.

For instance, you might consider that relationships with your family and friends are incredibly important, particularly after the cancer, but on thinking about it you might realize you don't spend much time on these things at all. So perhaps you can come up with a plan to connect more with these things that feel important. Alternatively, you might be spending lots of time and energy on things that, when you really think about it, don't feel that impor-tant at all. This kind of exercise can be helpful in guiding you and your person (if you do it together) about where you want to be heading, and how you can spend your time and energy in a way that feels meaningful.

11.

Why is everyone behaving like I'm back to normal?

Within weeks of being back at work it was like everyone had forgotten about the cancer. I was struggling to keep up with everything I needed to do, and whenever I tried to remind people about it, I just felt like they thought I was using it as an excuse.

Ming, 40 years old

As it turns out, people can often have very short memories. This is particularly true when people are recovering from cancer. For many people there will be visible signs of being unwell when going through treatment — particularly for those having chemotherapy and experiencing hair loss. When faced with someone who has obvious signs of being unwell, the people around will almost immediately act in a compassionate and caring way, and for the most part they will go out of their way to be helpful. However, as we have spoken about, it is often not when people are in treatment that they are struggling the most. For most patients, it is the period following treatment, when they are recovering and trying to make sense of what has just happened to them, that is the time they experience the most psychological difficulties.

Not the status quo

After treatment is finished, it may be that for the people around you, your world might start to look very 'normal' again. You might go back to work or study, start doing the things around the house you were doing before, and for the most part will start looking like you did previously. The physical scars and changes may be hidden from the outside world, except perhaps to intimate partners, and a shorter hairstyle might be the only obvious markers. Some of the residual difficulties people experience also tend to be quite invisible — things like fatigue, hormonal changes or pain — and many patients develop excellent skills at being able to mask these symptoms. There are likely to be people you meet now who know nothing about the cancer, or people who are known to you that you see infrequently who know nothing at all about what has happened in the past months. It is at this time that the expectations about what someone is able to manage can become skewed, as this invisibility of symptoms combined with the re-engagement in 'normal' activities often leads the people around you to assume that all is okay and the status quo has returned.

However, this is unlikely to be the case. Many of my patients speak to me about the frustration of people being oblivious to the difficulties they continue to experience, and can often feel that their support network is much more dismissive of where they are at. In the same way that patients experience 'cancer fatigue' (i.e. where they get sick of people only wanting to talk with them about cancer), their carer and support network can become fatigued about talking about it, and are so relieved that when the treatment ends and things can go back to 'normal' the cancer and its impact fades a little into the background. This may also be the time when the practical help might stop. Communities are generally very proactive and organized when someone is on treatment, with meals being delivered, tasks being done, kids being picked up, etc. But in the weeks after treatment stops it is likely this will cease as people assume it might not be needed any more. If prompted, family members and friends will likely reassure you that they haven't forgotten, but instead are just wanting to focus on moving forward. They may also assume that's what you want to happen as well.

'I'm okay'

One of the challenges inherent in this is that if you do not identify the difficulties you are experiencing, people are very unlikely to know that anything is wrong. Our general experiences in moving through the world tend to teach us that taking people at face value is a reasonable thing — most of the time, if people tell us they are okay, and they look like they are okay, and they are behaving as if they are okay, we assume that this is the case. Now of course, if you are faced with someone who is telling you they are okay but at the same time they have tears streaming down their face, you might not trust that this is the case in the same way. So if, in your situation, you are telling people that you are okay, and you are doing all the things you normally do, people will assume that all is okay.

And I bet I can guess what you are thinking. The people who know you really well should know that you're struggling, right? Well, some people will. And they might be the people who really surprise you. They might be the people you had not expected much support from, or people who maybe previously you hadn't been that close to. People who have had a difficult experience of cancer, or another significant illness or grief, will likely be much better placed to know how to support you, and as such they may be able to identify things that other people might be oblivious to. There might be some other people who you had/have high expectations of — good friends, perhaps, who you thought knew you better than anyone, but who can't seem to understand what you need from them. I don't want to provide excuses for people's behaviour; there might be people in your world who have truly behaved poorly in supporting you through all of this. But sometimes (or, in fact, most of the time) humans are very selfish creatures and we tend to spend quite a bit of time thinking about what it means for us when something happens. During cancer, people might feel ill equipped to help someone, feeling uncertain about what to do or how to do it. This can become even more pronounced at the end of treatment, when the cues about what needs to happen can be even less obvious.

Tell them what you need

Unfortunately, this is probably one of the areas where you need to tell people what you need. As nice as it would be to think that everyone in your world will continue to support you unprompted in the way that you need, let's assume this won't be the case. In order for that support to happen, it might be that you will need to point out that you need support. This of course can be really tricky for some people, and that is okay — it is a difficult thing to do.

First, think about what you actually need. You might have a sense that you are not feeling supported, but you need to work out in what way this isn't happening. Do you feel as if people have stopped asking you how you are? Are people assuming you can go back to working full time? Do people forget about the pain in your leg that slows you down when you have to walk a long way? Be specific about what the issue is.

The next part of the process is working out what you want people to do about the issue. Some things may be easier than others; for instance, asking someone to help carry your bags or deciding that you want to only work four days per week for now. Some might be a bit trickier, like needing a friend to check in with how you are going with the cancer stuff every now and then. If you have a specific thing that someone can do, it will make it easier for you to articulate it to them and make it easier for them to do it!

You might say to your boss, for example: 'The fatigue from the cancer treatment is still really difficult for me to manage. I have spoken with my doctors, who have told me it is likely to be around for a little while yet, and will improve gradually. I was hoping that to help me manage this I will be able to continue to work part time for the next couple of months.' Or you might say to a friend: 'I know that I'm doing better, but I am still really struggling with the after-effects of the cancer. I feel like lots of the people in my world have forgotten about it, and it would be great if you asked about it sometimes. There might be times when I have nothing to say, but then there will be times when I do.'

This dialogue might also be a nice opportunity to explore with your friends or family if they also have things they are not feeling supported with, and you might be able to do the same for them.

Not wanting to talk

The opposite problem can also present itself in this scenario, where you don't want to talk about the cancer at all, and the people around you will continually talk about it, or do everything for you, and try to stop you doing the things you know you can manage. The above steps work just as well here: work out what you need, and then work out how you are going to articulate this to the people around you.

There might be some people in your world who feel overwhelmed by the honesty in all of this, but if that is the case perhaps give them some time and space to process what you are asking of them, and then revisit again after a little time has passed.

As part of the cancer process generally, you might have made some decisions about who the important people in your world are, and it may be that some of the relationships you had before are unable to meet what you need right now. It may be that some of these will float off, and you could lose contact with people, but it is likely that you will also make new relationships or change some of your existing relationships to be much stronger as part of this process.

Summary of Part 2
Off treatment

Coming off treatment can feel as hard as, if not harder than, being on treatment. For many people, this will come as a bit of a shock, but with some preparation it is easier to make sense of this.

One of the most important parts of this is to give yourself time — all the things that await you in the world will still be waiting for you even if you take some time to make sense of everything that has happened. Remember, when you are in the process of treatment you will likely be just doing what you need to do to get through it; it's at the end that your brain catches up.

Here are the main points from Part 2.

Anxiety will turn up

It is normal for anxiety to come up for you at the end of treatment (even if you aren't someone who has been anxious before). This anxiety might look different from person to person, and it might be about lots of different things, but it is all based around uncertainty and your brain trying to understand what might happen next.

Know that there is a plan

We talked a lot in the first section about having a plan. The plan now is more theoretical — you don't need to know what the plan is exactly, but it is helpful to know that if your cancer returns, or if other unexpected things were to happen, your team will have a plan. They probably won't share it with you if you don't need to use it. Sometimes, though, knowing it exists is the helpful part.

It's okay not to have an epiphany

The experience of cancer will almost certainly change your life going forward, but it isn't likely to result in you making massive changes. In fact, I actively discourage you from making really big changes for at least six months after you finish treatment.

Clarify your values

The thing that might have changed after all this is that your values might have shifted, or you might feel that some things are less/more important than they were before. It is okay to spend some time working out where you sit with this and aligning your world with it.

Part 3

Living with advanced cancer

Rebecca had been feeling rubbish for a long time — she had no energy and was finding herself struggling to get through her busy days. She was trying to work as a teacher, but was finding that each day felt very long, and that she wasn't working at her best. She was only 40, and she couldn't believe that ageing was going to look like this for her. She had pains in her body that she was doing her best to ignore, but eventually when she went to the GP, she was sent off for lots of tests and investigations.

When her GP told her that he thought she had multiple myeloma, a disease of the plasma cells in her blood, she was a little bit relieved. All this time she had been convincing herself that it was all in her head, and that she was just tired. Having a diagnosis meant she could make sense of everything that was going on, but as more and more information came to her she began to be much more panicked about it.

Rebecca discovered when she met with her haematologist that her disease was manageable and treatable, but that she couldn't be cured. The myeloma would keep coming back, over and over again until it couldn't be treated any more. Her haematologist kept reassuring her that there were lots of treatments available for her, but also was using lots of words like 'aggressive' and 'difficult', which sent her into a bit of a spin whenever she heard them. When she started the treatment, she was surprised how well she felt; in fact, she felt better than she had for a long time. But her headspace felt much worse.

She couldn't make sense of knowing she would die from her disease. Even though she had been told it was likely she would live for a long time with the disease, possibly years, she found thoughts about how she would die rattling around in her mind almost constantly. She couldn't talk with anyone about them; no one in her world was likely to understand what it meant for her to be living with this. What made it more difficult was that she looked well. The treatment she was having didn't change the way that she looked at all. Rebecca was a very logical woman but couldn't understand how, when she was feeling better than she had felt in a long time, and looking better than she had in years, she could at the same time be dying.

Rebecca kept going to work and doing what she needed to do, but felt lost. The things that had felt like they had given her purpose in the past didn't feel the same any more, and she felt an incredible pressure that she should be doing things that were more meaningful than just going to work and going to the gym. She fantasized about packing up everything and going travelling around the world, but was too scared to be far away from the hospital in case something went wrong. She struggled to connect with her friends and family, who would tell her what was happening in their lives, all of which felt trivial and ridiculous and nothing compared to what it meant for her in her situation. She knew there was no point in talking with people about how she was feeling — she knew they couldn't possibly understand it.

The only thing that was helping her manage through this was knowing that she had a plan. She had spoken with her financial planner, and the lawyer. When she died, things would be organized, her friends and family would be her beneficiaries, and she felt good knowing they would be looked after. She had accumulated lots of assets and money over the years, but she noticed that she didn't really care much about it anymore. She found herself reading obsessively about how people make sense of living the end of their lives, and one of the things that kept coming through was that they found things that felt meaningful. She knew this would be the case for her too; she just couldn't quite work out what that thing was.

As a teacher, Rebecca had always liked routine, so she made sure that every day she was doing two things: one that made her feel good, and one that made her feel she was achieving something. She didn't know at the start what these things would be, but she found that over time, having these things in her life made her feel better. She loved walking in the bush near where she lived, so every afternoon after work she would walk around the pathway that led to the top of a hill. Some days when she was feeling really tired, she didn't make it to the top of the hill, but then other days she found herself at the top looking out over her town, feeling very grateful. The things that made her feel like she was achieving something changed from week to week. Sometimes she would be working her way through a book, sometimes she would be making something — a cake or a blanket — and at other times she would be doing a puzzle. Regardless, she found it very helpful to be able to look at something and know that she was making progress, even if it felt like small progress.

The thoughts about what would happen to her didn't go away, not by a long shot. They kept floating around in Rebecca's mind and would easily come to the front whenever she went to see her doctor or whenever she felt a new pain in her body. It took almost nothing to convince herself that the disease was back, and that this would be the time when it would all be over. But she knew that it didn't matter what she did, those thoughts would be around. She knew that she could fight with them, and stick her head in the sand to pretend it wasn't happening. But she knew that it wouldn't work. Rebecca's world had changed, and she couldn't go back to where she'd been. All she could do was find the things in her world that felt important, let the thoughts come and go, and be scared and anxious and worried sometimes.

12.

Living with advanced disease

I couldn't believe when the doctor sat down with me and told me that it was back. I had spent all that time doing treatment and all that I could, and it still came back anyway. Part of me felt broken in ways I can't describe, but then another part of me was desperate to do anything I could to fix it. Even though now, I don't truly believe I will be able to get rid of this.

Maeve, 60 years old

For some people, there will be the unfortunate moment where you might be told the cancer has returned. For others, they might have been told from the outset that they have disease that is advanced and unable to be cured. There are some slight differences in the processing of this information depending on whether you were diagnosed with advanced cancer or had treatment and your cancer has returned. The way people deal with these doesn't necessarily look different. But the path to it may.

Being diagnosed with advanced disease

Some people are told from the time of diagnosis that they have disease which has spread through their body. Generally, this means the cancer has moved from its original starting position (for instance the bowel) and has started growing in other places such as the lung, or bones. These other sites of disease might have been found because they had been causing you problems, like pain, or because the scans at the time of diagnosis might have shown other disease.

Almost all of my patients who are diagnosed with advanced disease talk about an accelerated processing of assuming that they will not be cured, and then trying to make sense of this. This doesn't necessarily mean they aren't hopeful that treatments will work, or that they decide they are going to die; but it often means they start thinking about the possibility that things might not be okay. Being diagnosed with advanced disease doesn't mean you won't survive the cancer, but it may mean that the landscape of treatment and the ongoing ability to 'get rid of it' completely might look different than for someone who is diagnosed with a local cancer. This is a difficult space to sit in, and for many of the people I see it will take them a long time to make some sense of what it means to have a diagnosis of advanced cancer.

Just as we talked about in the section around diagnosis, you might feel overwhelmed, fearful, angry, sad or relieved. Or you might feel all these things together. It's hard to make sense of what it means to have this kind of diagnosis. Hopefully, as we work through this section you might be able to find some strategies that will help make it feel just a little more manageable.

The cancer came back

When you hear this news it may feel like it has come from nowhere, and it might smash you in the guts so hard that you think you will never stand up again. Or (and this does happen for some people) you might find that the cancer returning allows you some relief, in that the thing you had been so fearful of for so long has arrived, and now you know you can do something with it.

Regardless of how you feel about it, quite universally most people speak about their experience of the second time around in the context of how different it feels. It might feel more intense, or it might feel like the stakes are higher, or it might be accompanied with some worries and thoughts about how you could possibly manage to make it through treatment again. It's pretty likely that those thoughts and worries about mortality and what might happen to you will reappear at the front of your mind, and it will probably be hard to distract yourself from them. You might find you don't sleep and eat for a couple of days, and the numbness you felt first time around might be feeling more real again. The shock and worry about the return of the cancer might look quite like that initial diagnosis time or it may look quite different. Regardless, a similar pattern might occur when you work out what the plan is going to be, and you might find you will feel more settled in yourself.

Almost all patients tell me that when the cancer returns it feels different. There seems to be a shift for people around what the cancer returning means. It may contain more concrete thoughts about what it would mean not to survive the cancer in a way that you may not have processed before. The return of the cancer doesn't mean you won't survive your cancer, but it might mean that the landscape of treatment and the ongoing ability to 'get rid of it' completely looks different than what it did before. The urge to get more information from the internet might pick up again, but I would advise staying away from this as it is likely to do nothing other than terrify you and give you information that is likely to be out of date and not helpful for you. Instead, ask your doctors about what is happening.

So in both cases, what do I do?

Some of the words that come along after this might feel hard to read, and if it doesn't feel like the right time to read them, that is okay — you can come back later if you feel you need to.

I am willing to bet that there are some pretty difficult thoughts appearing for you. And most of them are probably grouped together as the 'worst-case scenario'.

It wouldn't surprise me if you told me that after you got the news about your cancer you started to have some thoughts about dying. It makes sense that this is the thing that has started to play on your mind. It might have been prompted by your doctors telling you that the cancer isn't fixable, or maybe you have known other people where this is the case. The reality for many people who have their cancer return is that they will die from their cancer. But that doesn't mean everyone, and it doesn't mean that it will happen. Some people will have their cancer return, have further treatment and then not have any other issues again. With the changing nature of treatments, there are some people who will live with advanced cancer for many years, and live relatively normal lives.

However, regardless of all of the above, you are likely to be worried about the future, and as such you will likely be more worried about whether or not you will die from this. It makes sense that this will be amplified and might shift and change as you settle in to the plan for the next steps in treatment. These are hard thoughts to carry with you, and you are probably working pretty hard to try to get rid of them.

Allow the thought to be there

Paradoxically, sometimes one of the best things you can do with this worst-case scenario thinking is to be present to it and allow it to be there, because in all likelihood the presence of this worry and concern will be a bit of a constant going forward in your life. It might fade or shift a little over time, but in the days and weeks following the news this thought about what is going to happen to you is likely to occupy many of your sleeping and waking moments. And, in actual fact, trying to get rid of it is likely to be as successful as that old idea of not thinking of the pink elephant. You know the one, where someone tells you not to think of a pink elephant. I am willing to bet as you are reading this you are picturing a pink elephant, and perhaps now it is dancing.

No matter how much you try not to worry or think about this stuff, it is likely to be present and in your world, so allowing it to be there and working out how to manage it is probably going to be the key. This is one of those things that is easy for me to say and in all likelihood much harder for you to do. For lots of us, the idea of letting our worries and fears about our mortality be around will feel like an overwhelming tide that you can't do anything to swim against. Or for some, the idea of allowing this to be present is not unlike inviting it in, and you may think that by thinking about it you are jinxing yourself that this will happen to you. However, there is a difference between being able to allow the thoughts that will appear anyway to be present and not get too caught up with them, and assuming that any thought about this at all will lead to the thing you are thinking coming true. In my experience there is no connection between thinking about this stuff and whether it will happen. But if you try to stop yourself thinking these worst-case scenario thoughts it is likely you will feel completely overwhelmed.

As we have talked about in Chapter 4, to manage these thoughts first acknowledge that they are okay to be there. It might be that for you, you can find different words, but sometimes the simplest way of doing this is to tell yourself, 'It's okay that these thoughts are there; it is a way of my brain doing its job and trying to look after me.' Often there is a fear that letting the thoughts be around at all will mean they will run and take over, but it usually goes the other way. When you can identify why the thoughts are turning up and are more comfortable with their presence, you save the energy that it takes to fight against them.

Struggling and the tug of war

Acceptance and Commitment Therapy (ACT for short) uses the analogy of struggle. I have borrowed the below example from Russ Harris's *The Happiness Trap*.

Picture yourself standing on the end of a tug-of-war rope, and your thoughts about this worst-case scenario are on the other end. Most of us will spend lots of time pulling tightly on the rope to make sure that the thoughts don't win (or in this case, it might be that if you fight hard enough against the idea of the worst case, you might be able to think it won't happen). Instead, the only real way to win the tug of war is to drop the rope. Can you imagine that idea? If you stop struggling with these ideas and holding onto the rope so tightly, and simply let it go, the thoughts at the other end of the rope are likely to fall solidly onto their bums, and you will be left standing up. The thoughts haven't gone away — they will still be standing there at the end of the rope, trying to get your attention and wanting you to engage with them.

Without realizing it, you might pick up the rope lots of times, and find yourself struggling away with them again, but that's okay; you can notice that and then notice the ways you can stop struggling with them. If you see that they are just thoughts, and your brain will keep throwing them up, and it's okay that they are there, all of a sudden they may feel a little more manageable. Note, they probably won't be pleasant, and at times you will get caught up in them, but they will stay with you and it's okay that they are there.

There might be some thoughts that are helpful in getting important things done. For instance, if the information from your doctor implores you to organize your will or other legal documents it is worth doing that (we will talk about this more in Chapter 14). Sometimes doing these practical things — even if you don't end up needing them — will help you to feel more settled in yourself. This will also include things like managing pain, taking the medications you need to, or attending appointments and treatment. All of this will likely help you manage the demands of everything that is happening.

How long have I got?

Many people feel conflicted in even considering asking this question of their doctors. If you know that your cancer has returned, your next logical step could be, as it is for many people, to start planning and trying to anticipate the worst (in an attempt to feel prepared if it were to happen), which might mean seeking information about what timeframe you may be looking at. We know that, on the whole, doctors are not very good at predicting this. And giving you specific information that might be incorrect is likely to be psychologically very unhelpful.

One of the more helpful ways of looking at this is to think about what you want to know and why. For some people, having an idea of the prognosis is linked to feeling less anxious or worried, or feeling like they have more of a plan. Would you want your doctor to be really upfront with you, and tell you in no uncertain terms if they were confident that you were deteriorating and likely to die? Or would you perhaps want them to withhold this information so that you could be ignorant of what might be happening for you? There is no right or wrong way of doing this — some people will have a preference for one way over another, but many people will sit in the middle, and equally it might be a space that changes over time.

Talking with your team about what you would want to know in this situation allows them to help give you this information (if there is information to be given). It is worth thinking through what it would mean if you opted to have this information: would it allow you to feel that you could plan things better? Or would you likely feel overwhelmed by it? Conversely, what does it look like to not have that information: would your anxiety actually be higher as you feel like you don't know what is going on? This is a really complex decision to make, and I recommend that if you are struggling with it, talk with someone about it. Sometimes talking this through will actually allow you to think about what you want or need in a way that feels safe. One of my colleagues, Iris, often asks her patients the question, 'How would you want to live your life if you knew the prognosis? What changes would you make?' Thinking about it in this way might mean you are able to think about the things you value and how you might be able to engage with those things right now.

Telling others

People often communicate to me that this information can feel really isolating. It may be that people have even less capacity to understand what your world looks like, or they may assume you will need things that you might not.

It's helpful to again revisit the idea of what you need from people and then tell them, because it is very unlikely they will be able to guess. You may find yourself feeling as if you are walking around in the world with the knowledge that you have limited time, which will change all the ways that you make sense of what you do and what feels important, but will also have a cascade effect onto what other people are doing around you.

Making sense of all of this information will take a bit of time and practice. Unless someone has been in the same situation as you it is unlikely that they will understand, and as a result you might find yourself feeling alone on a desert island, waiting for a boat to arrive to help you back.

13.

Finding your purpose and meaning:
part 3

I thought I had started to make sense of what it meant to be living with this whole life-limiting illness thing - but sometimes it just comes and knocks me off my feet.
Brian, 64 years old

It's hard to imagine that there would be another 'new normal' to adjust to isn't it?

You have already had to manage the impact of your world being turned upside down when the cancer arrived for the first time, and then again when you finished treatment and perhaps found that the normal you were seeking was not what you thought it would be. Or perhaps you were hoping the cancer that looked like it had gone away might stay away. Or maybe in the last couple of months or weeks you've finished treatment and started planning what the next stage of your life might look like; you may have even started to put the memory of the cancer to the back of your mind (although I suspect it hasn't fallen off the radar completely). Then, in what probably felt like a split second, you hear the words that you feared.

The cancer has come back. Or perhaps it never went away.

It might have snuck back without you knowing anything about it, or it might have announced itself loudly back into your world. Either way, I would assume that you felt completely sideswiped by its reappearance. If you were really anxious about the return, you may have found some relief in the certainty of it returning, which might feel counter-intuitive, but often (particularly with something that can feel as difficult to manage as this) having some certainty allows you to start to make some plans. However, the sense of certainty will almost undoubtedly be overshadowed by incredible fear, sadness, terror or any of those other emotions that might pop up at this time.

This means that the emotions in themselves might feel normal, or they might feel like the body you cannot quite get comfortable in. You might feel able to open yourself to being present to the experience of the fear and worry, or your instinct might be to take your head and plant it firmly in the sand. Both of these strategies have some utility, and you might oscillate between them as you work out what you need, and when you need it. Many people describe to me the sense of knowing that things have changed when the cancer comes back, and that the feeling of time pressure and not knowing how much time is left amplifies things in a way it may not have before. This can be the case, even if you don't truly believe that you will die from the cancer, and in fact may occur even if people around you are telling you that the cancer is still fixable. There is something in the mechanism of it returning again that makes it much harder to disconnect from the sense of mortality that may have come up first time around.

FINDING MEANING   **OVERWHELMED**

Practicalities

The practicalities of normal in themselves might look quite different. If you have been told you will need treatment again, you may find yourself much less likely to want to juggle treatment with work or other things. You may think that if time feels more precious, there are many things you'd been doing before that you no longer want to do; these could range from simple and small to big and complex. Alternatively, it might be that more than ever the structure of going to work and having to be organized to face the day everyday feels really important and the thing that helps balance out all the other things that might play out in the cancer side of your world. Or perhaps the urge to do treatment this time around feels less urgent, and you may feel more ambivalent about what you should do next — this could lead you to explore other therapies or doctors that you had never even considered before.

Immediately after finding out the cancer has returned, many of my patients speak about uncertainty and feeling like the world has been turned upside down again. But coincidently they may find they experience a clarity they didn't have in the past. This clarity can be about lots of things, but it is rarely like an epiphany; instead, it is usually much more about the smaller everyday things that ultimately make up our lives.

> It was like all of a sudden my life became more like a tunnel, and lots of things just fell away the second that I heard that it had returned. All of the things I promised that I would do after the last time became the things that I actually needed to do now.
>
> Jen, 45 years old

Just as we have spoken about before, the meaning and importance of things will of course change in this space. We generally exist under the very false pretence that nothing will ever take our time away, but of course (and I don't need to explain this to you!) things happen that do challenge that notion of never-ending time. From the time we are very small children, we have a knowledge (and to some extent an understanding) that we are going to die. However, we are rarely ever conscious or aware of this, instead pushing it far into the back of our brains and pretending it won't happen. But for you right now, I am willing to bet that the connection around this is much more real and salient, and as a result I imagine you also find yourself being much more connected to the sense that this is a time to just get things done, and do the things that matter.

Dealing with your mortality

First up, I need to say that there is absolutely no right way to do this. I have spoken to thousands of people over the years, and everyone approaches these ideas of existential identity and making sense of their own mortality in very different ways.

However, there have been some themes that come through.

A clarity about what is important

As I alluded to earlier, this is about taking the moments that feel meaningful and important and removing the things from your life that perhaps don't feel so important. Now, I am putting a caveat around this: not everything in your life can feel meaningful. You will still need to take the garbage out, feed the kids and endure boring conversations, just as you would have had to do before. It is almost impossible to live in a space where everything is full of meaning. It might just be that, now, you direct most of your energy to the things that feel more important.

A move towards values

We have spoken about values as we have worked through this book, but it is often at this time in people's lives where they can solidify the things they value in a way they might have struggled with in the past.

Values can fit in to a couple of main domains, but generally are related to family/friends/connections; yourself and the things that feel important to you; your community; spiritual beliefs; and how you spend your time (recreation or leisure). There can be much more complex versions of thinking about this, but like most things in life, it seems that generally the simple things work really well. So, these things may already be really obvious to you, or maybe you are struggling to work out what you value right now. Either way, it might be worth thinking about the domains above, and deciding if they are relevant to you (some may really obviously not be, and some might feel incredibly important). Then when you have an idea of what the important ones might be, it's worth asking the question, how would I know if I am living according to my values? How could you engineer your world to make sure you are doing the things that feel important? If you are experiencing lots of physical symptoms it's not likely that your underlying values will have changed, but the ways you move towards your values in your day-to-day life might have to change — so if this is the case, perhaps consider how you can change what you normally do to help manage this so you can continue to live in a way that is important to you. For instance, if one of your key values is spending time with your kids but you're normally quite hands-on and active with them, perhaps you need to shift some of your activities to be gentler, such as doing a puzzle or building a Lego castle. The important thing is that you are still acting in line with your values.

The way you measure day-to-day success might change

By success, I don't mean whether you live or die, but your sense of meaning and purpose. The things that felt important and the way you measured success before cancer likely looked different than when you finished treatment, and now this may have changed again. If your physical condition has changed it is likely that, just by the nature of the energy you have and the situation you are in, the things you find achievable each day might look quite different.

It is important to be kind to yourself when measuring success. Many patients find themselves wedded to the idea that the new normal will continue to look very similar to the old normal, forgetting that as a consequence of where they are physically it is likely to look different.

Less tolerance for people

This isn't all people, of course, but it does make perfect sense that if you felt less connected to particular people during all the cancer stuff this will continue to be the case as you now navigate through the next part. However, you may also find that overall your capacity and tolerance for everyone might be less. This ties in with the time pressure we talked about before. Most of my patients who might be facing the end of their lives, or feel that they have limited time, don't have much desire to engage in things like small talk, or talk about things that feel like they don't matter (that is, that they feel they don't matter to *them*; they might be able to identify that they matter quite a lot to the people who want to talk with them).

You might find yourself getting irritated with the people who are closest to you, and it may be for reasons you can't quite put your finger on; you just know that they are more irritating.

Gratefulness in a way you haven't experienced before

Sometimes in the landscape of the cancer and all of this uncertainty, the smaller things in life take on a significance you may not have noticed before. For instance, waking up in the morning may feel more significant than it had in the past, or you may experience gratitude at being able to sit in the sunshine and feel the warmth on your shoulders. It's easy in the cancer space to get stuck just thinking about the things that aren't going well, or the unpleasant things you need to endure. I suspect, though, there are things to be grateful for, and it is worth acknowledging them when they come to you (have a look at Chapter 24 on gratitude).

You might question the meaning of all of this

As we mentioned before, our sense of mortality can often be a funny thing

— and we are often disconnected from it. When the cancer returns many people start to ask questions of themselves that they wouldn't normally — why this has happened to them, for instance, or what the purpose of life itself is. This is, of course, normal when you're facing your own mortality, and as a result you might find that in asking yourself these questions the way you look at the world starts to change. The tricky thing is that these thoughts are a little bit like Alice's rabbit hole and very quickly can become overwhelming.

It's important to make a distinction between thinking about some of these bigger-picture existential concepts and getting completely caught up in examining whether your life has any purpose. If you are thinking about the latter and feeling hopeless in your situation, it is important that you make some connections with a health professional to help you make sense of this, as it might be a sign that your thinking is becoming a little more depressed.

Many philosophers have dedicated their entire lives to making sense of all this existential stuff and, as far as I know, no one has been able to find an answer. You might find an answer that works for you, and that answer might be to not think about it too much, or it might be to think about it lots. But whichever way it goes, it is probably worth being cognisant that spending too much time thinking about this stuff ultimately means that you are probably missing out on doing some other things that also feel important.

There may be some unexpected things that come up which are not in this list

That's really the nature of this: I can almost never predict what it is that people will struggle with, and what will sit well. Whatever comes up is probably there for a reason, so notice it, allow it to be present, and explore what may come from it.

A new routine

Despite the upheaval that the news of the cancer returning can bring, it is likely that after a while you will find yourself settling back into a routine of sorts — perhaps a slightly different routine than you had previously, but it is likely to come back. As we mentioned earlier, it is almost impossible to do meaningful things all the time, and it is almost impossible to think for any significant period of time solely about the cancer returning and what that might mean. Instead, it's common for getting settled into a routine with some kind of structure to be comforting and helpful, and it's likely you will move towards this.

> I just couldn't be bothered with work anymore, but I could sit for hours and draw, just like I did when I was younger.
> Julia, 45 years old

What you need as time changes might look really different. Sometimes, as your world starts to feel smaller because of treatment or perhaps where you are psychologically, it makes sense that the things you need might be much more simple, and you might find you are content to do things that would normally not feel enough at all, such as watching movies and television. Or you might find yourself seeking and craving a really substantial project to fill the sense of purpose you need. Either option is fine, as long as you are listening to what you need and what your body needs.

You might find yourself being pulled and torn in lots of different directions right now, by people who no doubt only want the best for you. But it is pretty likely they have not stood in the position you are standing in. This is one of those times in life when you can truly make the decisions and spend your time how you want to spend it.

TIPS FOR CARERS:
Dealing with advanced cancer

Sometimes cancers can't be fixed. This is tough stuff to hear, and you are likely to find yourself spinning into some panic and anxiety, or you might feel as if you can't really make sense of it at all. Regardless, this information will have an impact on you, the person you are caring for, the things you do or prioritize and even on people who are more removed from the situation. As the carer, it might even be you who communicates this kind of news to other people in your network — which is a really tough job to have.

How well your person is might determine in some way how you start to process it. For instance, if your person is very unwell, you have seen a deterioration in them and they have symptoms they haven't had before, it might be much easier to contemplate them not getting better than if your person is very well and their cancer was an incidental finding on a scan and they are absolutely asymptomatic. Also, if you feel you have a good understanding of what is happening medically, and a grasp on why the cancer can't be fixed, it might help you feel more able to process the information yourself and also to communicate it when you need to. If you feel like you don't have a good handle on it, it is reasonable to chat with the oncologist or specialist and work out what it is that you don't understand. It sounds simple, but it can make the process a little easier if you feel like you know what the plan is and what the reasoning is behind it.

This news might mean that you and your person have conversations you have never had before. These conversations are really tough and sometimes confronting. They may be around things like wills or estates, or funerals and decision making. For most patients, doing these things brings a sense of relief, even if it is really tough to do. It gives some control at a time when everything probably feels pretty unclear.

Generally, a good way of thinking about all these things is to focus on the short term rather than too far ahead. It sounds easier to do than it is, but whenever you think too far into the future that's where the uncertainty lives, and trying to anticipate what might happen next will probably just make you feel anxious. In this kind of situation, our brains automatically try to think through every future possibility. I am sure that by now you have worked out that there isn't really an end point for this, and so your brain will just keep spinning and spinning to find an answer (and it probably won't find one!). This process can be exhausting, can impact what you are able to focus on and get done, and is really hard to contain. Instead, it's better to try to stay focused on the here and now. Think about the next hour or so, and maybe even the next day, but just try to keep it there.

Confronting challenging ideas and thoughts

When your person's cancer can't be fixed it might bring up a bunch of challenging and confronting concepts for you. You may have had some experience with death in the past, or conversely this might be the first time you have had to grapple with the idea of losing someone you care deeply about. Being around people who are facing their own mortality may also mean you question some of your own thoughts and beliefs about these concepts. It might be a tough thing for you to find other people to talk to about this. If you are finding it really difficult to make sense of this stuff, I would recommend that you seek out the support of a professional — they won't likely have the answers but they may help clarify some things and give you space to talk about where you are.

There may be some unique challenges for you in trying to navigate this situation as a carer, particularly if the news of advanced disease comes after lots of previous treatment and uncertainty. You might already be feeling exhausted when this news comes, and it may be tough for you to think about how you can manage this next piece when you don't have the energy. Perhaps being on autopilot has got you through so far: going through the motions of diagnosis, treatment and maybe even having some time when you felt as if you were starting to make sense of things again. And then you have been hit with this news. Most people acknowledge, for both carers and patients, that the second time around feels more discombobulating than the first diagnosis. Partially, this is due to the sense of not knowing how they can face doing it all again, particularly if now the outcome might feel more uncertain.

You might also find yourself thinking about what it would be like if your person did die, and what it would be like for you afterwards. Sometimes these thoughts might come in sadness and grief, or they may come in frustration at the end of a long day, or when times are really difficult. These are kind of taboo thoughts, right? This isn't the stuff you talk about with people, but almost every carer I have ever met has thought about this at some time or another. These thoughts might be fleeting or they might hang around for a bit. I like to think of them like problem solving: if these thoughts are coming from sadness, it is driven by your brain trying to protect you. It's trying to anticipate and prepare you for something that would be really difficult to manage. Of course, these thoughts don't change the difficult reality if your person was to die, but our brains always try to help us out about this stuff. If the thoughts are coming from frustration, or exhaustion, or overwhelm, it is a similar idea, just a bit of a different function. At these times, your brain is trying to give you options, almost like an escape. This is a really difficult time, and a really difficult thing to make sense of, so your brain is fantasizing about a time when it may be different. Neither of these situations (or any others that come up around this theme) mean that you want your person to die. They are just thoughts coming from a brain that is trying to help you when you are in a really difficult space.

14.

Planning and decision-making (even if you don't need it!)

Until I made the appointment with the solicitor it just felt like something was hanging over my head — like I needed to get it done. It was hard to do, but when I did, I was relieved. I didn't need to think about it anymore.

Cal, 48 years old

As humans we like a plan — we have talked about this as we have weaved our way through the book. One of the times when the sense of a plan can feel particularly important is when we think there is a likelihood that something bad will happen. Almost all of my patients who have found themselves in this situation talk about the deep sense of need and urgency to make sure all the practical things are covered — things like wills, power of attorney documents as well as some of the legacy stuff, such as leaving things for particular people or writing letters.

Of course, this is difficult stuff to do. Even when things are going well, most people struggle to attend to these tasks, with the mere thought of what they mean being quite an existential challenge. If things are going less well, many people find the idea of doing these tasks completely overwhelming. However, the other side of this equation is that people often feel compelled to 'sort these things out' just in case anything happens. Although these tasks are hard to do, people generally feel relieved when completed, and they become the things you don't have to worry about anymore. This works particularly well for things like wills. At some stage we all need to have one, and once it is done, it is done; even if nothing bad happens in the immediate future it is something you don't have to think about going forward. One of the hallmarks of western society is that we often actively avoid thinking about our own death, and the avoidance of attending to these documents can be an extension of this. Most of my patients, prior to doing them, describe thinking over and over again about needing to do them and feeling a sense of pressure that they haven't. They then feel the pressure has been taken off afterwards.

Leaving a legacy

Legacy-leaving is a slightly more complex practical task. Everyone has different ideas about legacy and what's important: some people will feel compelled to leave concrete things like letters or gifts for people to remember them by, while others may consider the very act of having children or some other meaningful work as their legacy. Either way it is likely you will be thinking about some of these things (even though they are likely to be really difficult to think about at times). This is your brain trying to help you out again — it is thinking 'Well, if something happens to me I want to be remembered and I want to leave my mark on the world, so how can I do that?' Of course, our immediate people will hold a strong memory and recollection of us when we are gone; but for others we are likely to fade, so this work around legacy can mean that you feel assured there are concrete pieces of you out there in the world.

Almost everyone I meet talks about wanting to do this work, but almost no one does. Why? Because it is really hard work to do. It is confronting and scary and often sad if it forces you into thinking about a future without you in it. But even though it is difficult, the work around legacy usually feels important for people, so working out how to do it is often the key. Note, these steps won't make it not be difficult, but will hopefully give you some guidelines to help it feel more manageable.

Work out what you want your legacy to be, or what you want to focus on

Looking at all the possible options for how you might be remembered is likely to be completely overwhelming. So think about the things and people that matter to you; think about how you would like to be remembered by those closest to you. Is your legacy about people (leaving notes or things to the people you care about) or the wider community (leaving things to a project or community organization, sharing your knowledge or skills in some way)?

Start small

I have had patients over time who start out with colossal tasks, such as leaving their young children a handwritten card for each birthday until they turn 30 or writing letters to everyone in their world. This is a fast path to burnout and won't get any of the work finished.

Instead, perhaps pick one or two things and start with those. In the above example, that might mean writing cards for the eighteenth and 21st birthdays, or it might mean writing something for the five people closest to you. If after these you want to do more, of course that is fine, but make it manageable so that you get what you want done rather than being completely overwhelmed and stuck.

Expect that doing this will make you feel sad, and as a result you will probably avoid doing it

As strange as it sounds, you should probably be a bit opportunistic about doing this difficult work when you feel reasonably okay physically (this is not the thing to try to do when you feel really exhausted or in pain). It is also good to have something nice to do afterwards. Sitting down to work this stuff out will be pretty emotional and it's likely to be quite exhausting as well, so having something pleasant and rejuvenating to do afterwards is probably not a bad plan.

As with writing a will and other difficult things, you are likely to feel relieved when it is done, and completing it may well leave you with a sense of peace that this thing that feels so important is sorted out.

Approaching the end of life

This section might feel tough to read. It may not feel like the right time to read it, or it may feel like the thing you want to do. Either way, it's okay to just notice what comes up for you and be present to those emotions. This is hard stuff to make sense of, but it may be that by reading through you find some reassurance for things you are struggling with.

If you have been told you are going to die from your cancer this is horrible news to hear. Whether you were expecting to hear this news or it came as a complete shock, one of the most important things to do is allow yourself time to grieve. This grief will look different from person to person, but is often about making sense of the idea of you no longer being present in the world, as well as grieving the loss of your own future and also your role in other people's futures.

We have spoken lots about the importance of feeling like you have a plan, and at this time in your life it might feel like there are some really big parts to plan for. These might include the following.

A funeral

Some people find comfort in organizing their own funeral or celebration of their life. At times it might feel appropriate to have a funeral before someone dies, with an opportunity to have a great party with everyone they want to see in one room. Other people can't stand the idea. Many people will be quite absolute about these things and rationalize that there is no point in planning things they won't be a part of. Either way, it's important that you talk with the people close to you about what you want — this is partially for you, but much more for the people around you so they feel that they are able to honour whatever wishes you may have.

What the end of life might look like

You may have questions about what the end of your life will look like. Depending on your situation this might be something that is easy to predict, or not. But perhaps the more important thing is seeking reassurance from your team about whatever you are worried about, and understanding their plan to manage it. In my experience, people are generally worried about pain and discomfort, and these are things that can be managed, so speaking with your team about this is an important thing to do.

Where you want to die

You might have really strong feelings about this, and may have thought a lot about where you want your final time to be. But many people don't ever give this much thought. It's important to have open conversations with your family, the people you want around you at the end of your life, and your treating team.

For most people I work with, as they approach the end of their lives their world starts to feel much smaller. Things very quickly solidify around what they feel is important, and what they want to spend time thinking about. Very quickly this news may shift what conversations you want to have, what you want to eat, who you want to spend time with, and what you worry about. Things that before might not have felt particularly significant may give you pleasure in a way you have not previously experienced — for instance, sitting outside in the sunshine can sometimes feel like a very important and magical thing, whereas having to contemplate decisions about what you have for dinner may not. This of course will vary from person to person, and you might be surprised by what feels important to you now.

Summary of Part 3
Living with advanced cancer

This section has focused on what it means psychologically to have a cancer that is advanced (spread to other parts of your body than the original tumour, or you may have been diagnosed with a cancer that is life-limiting). This is a hard space to sit in, and many patients struggle with making sense of lots of complex and existential ideas when they are faced with ideas around their mortality.

Here are a few things that might help you navigate through.

You might feel lost

It's likely you have not thought about your mortality (or maybe not even thought much about the future in general), so you might find thoughts about this quite confronting. In these moments it might feel hard to connect with things that would normally feel good. Or you might question whether there is meaning in some of the things that you are doing.

Time might feel funny

Inherent in thinking about the future is that you might start thinking about the meaning of time differently. You might feel the pressure of having to do lots of things that feel important and meaningful; or conversely, you may feel overwhelmed by not quite knowing what to do. If this happens, it helps to stop and think about your values and what feels really important. This is almost always the way of working through this — do the things that feel most meaningful, and allow yourself to let go of the things that don't.

Have a plan

Having a plan at this time might feel even more important. The plan might be around your daily activities, or it might be about what you want to happen to your belongings if you are to die (and perhaps lots of places in between). Thinking about these things means you will be able to manage the uncertainty of the future much better (although the uncertainty will continue to creep in from time to time).

Part 4

The psychology part: How can you manage all of this?

Peter is 53 years old. He has always worked. Always. He remembers getting his first job at fifteen and has only had four sick days since then. The jobs he has had have never been kind to his body, and he has always had aches all over. So when he started to have a pain in his back, he didn't think too much of it. Until he ended up with a cough that wouldn't go away.

His wife Margie sent him off to the GP, and even though he didn't think it was anything, the GP sent him off for an X-ray. There it was, plain as day: a big tumour in his lung that was causing the pain in his back. The GP said it was probably the cigarettes he used to have when he was younger. He had stopped, though, years ago. He was told he would need to have chemotherapy to see if they could shrink the tumour.

Peter had known some blokes who'd had chemo before, and it knocked them around, so he was a bit worried about it. But when Margie tried to talk with him about it, he said that he was fine.

When he had the first dose of chemotherapy, Peter was surprised that he felt as good as he did. He had been worried about the nausea and vomiting, but he didn't have any of that. The problem was, though, that because he had planned to be sick, and he wasn't, he was sitting around at home driving himself mad with worry. He couldn't remember the last time he had spent this much time at home. He just didn't know what to do with himself. He tried to watch television and do some reading, but he couldn't focus as he would like to. The dog was following him around, but he wasn't sure whether he was able to walk her. He tried to think about what he would normally do when he was at home on the weekends: he would normally be outside in the garden, spending time with the kids and Margie, or at the pub with his mates. But they were all at work.

Peter hadn't really told people much about what was going on. The guys at the workshop knew because he wasn't around, but when he went to visit they didn't ask too much about it. All he was thinking about was the cancer and worrying about the next treatment. Even though he felt well, the second that he felt any twinge in his body any-where, he was sure it must be these horrible side effects starting that everyone talked about.

Peter couldn't believe how much it all affected him. He found him-self feeling really scared and alone, even though his wife and mates were around. He was spending more and more time by himself, which he knew wasn't a very helpful thing to be doing, but he couldn't be bothered to get out and see people. He had never really been one to think too much about things, but he couldn't turn his brain off. And it wasn't telling him helpful stuff; it was all about the cancer and how bad everything was. He felt irritable with everything — it didn't matter what Margie did, it was the wrong thing, and he was snapping at her all the time. Problem was, he knew it wasn't anything she was doing, and then he'd beat himself up for talking to her badly.

He didn't much get the point of doing all of the treatment and things if he was just going to live like this — stuck in his house, staring at the walls and thinking of all the terrible things in his world. He knew that it wasn't that bad, but he couldn't get it out of his head. It didn't seem to matter what he did.

The kids were worried about Peter; he could see it when they were around. Loule, the youngest one, took him out fishing and they didn't catch a thing, but Peter noticed that he felt better when he came back. Must have been the fresh air. And while he was out there fishing, cold sand underneath his toes, he didn't think about the cancer once.

15.

Mood vs treatment

As the cycles went on I noticed a change, I just didn't bounce back the way that I had before. I would be feeling better after the chemo, but I still did not want to leave the house or talk to anyone. I was just locked away in my little flat wanting it all to be done.

Meera, 35 years old

A common question I am asked is, 'How would I know if I am depressed?' The side effects of some cancer treatments can mirror depression, adding a layer of complexity to this question. In this chapter, we'll first look at depression on its own, and then at what that looks like when you are being treated for cancer.

Depression

Depression can be a bit of a funny character — it has a habit of sneaking up on people and appearing as if from nowhere, and for those who have been depressed in the past the familiar feelings of overwhelm, hopelessness and negativity can come knocking at the door in the least opportune times.

Depression for most people will have a couple of common features. Typically, there will be few signs that appear along the way, but it is often not until the symptoms become really significant that people realize they are feeling quite depressed. Depression can occur in the context of a big life event, such as a significant relationship break-up, changes in lifestyle or situation, or it may occur due to changes in brain chemistry. Sometimes it will be a combination of both.

So, how would you know if you are depressed?

Cancer complicates the whole picture around depression, so let's take this out of the equation for a second (don't worry, we will come back to it in a moment). There are a few hallmark signs for depression, although it is important to note that everyone's experience will look a little bit different.

Withdrawal

Many people with depression describe a sense of wanting or needing to reduce their activities, including the things that normally provide them with pleasure. This can be multifactorial and may accompany feelings of anxiety or overwhelm when trying to do activities that might normally feel quite manageable, such as catching up with a friend for coffee.

Low motivation

When people start to do less, the natural pattern is that they then want to do less; then they do even less and want to do even less. Do you see where this is heading? This sometimes results in even simple tasks feeling completely overwhelming, and people will consequently not be able to manage them. In addition to this, though, the nature of depression is that you are likely to have some very negative thoughts that will accompany anything that happens, and you will beat yourself up for not doing the things you would normally be able to manage.

Negative thoughts

This is one of the most common and difficult parts of being depressed.

People often describe a barrage of thoughts swirling around all the time, most of which are very negative in nature. It's the thoughts that come when you least expect it, and hit people pretty hard. Thoughts that tell you that you are not good enough or question why people would want to spend time with you; sometimes they will take you down a path you don't want to go down, like questioning whether you should be around at all.

Often when people are experiencing these kinds of thoughts it's hard to get a sense of what is real and not, so people may not make good decisions. If you are having these kind of thoughts, I would advise that you seek professional help immediately in managing them.

Sense of hopelessness about the future

In combination with the negative thoughts, it can be difficult for people to feel positive about the future, which can become a process of feeling completely overwhelmed and unable to picture what any future might look like. For some people this can include thoughts about ending their life. Again, if you are having these kinds of thoughts, I would advise that you seek professional help immediately in managing them.

Changes in the way you feel or interact with other people

Often, people who are feeling depressed describe feeling flat or depressed. However, as we talked about before, depression can be a bit of a tricky beast, so it might not always look like this. Lots of people describe feeling irritable and frustrated all the time, or unable to tolerate things that they normally would (like noises). They may feel guilty about everything (including things they know they don't need to feel guilty about) or they may have difficulty in making decisions. These things in themselves are not enough to describe depression, but if they are occurring with other issues as above it might indicate that your mood has changed.

Physical changes

People may experience changes in their sleep and appetite — either sleeping or eating too much, or sleeping or eating too little. They may feel fatigued all the time, or feel that their minds aren't working as well as they normally would. Sometimes they may have stomach upsets or headaches.

Add in the complexity of cancer

As I mentioned before, the above list of symptoms is what we would expect to see in someone without cancer (or another significant health problem) if they were depressed. But the picture gets a lot more complex when we add cancer and its treatments into the mix.

The side effects of cancer treatments can often mirror depression, with a few very important differences. So let's look at that same list of symptoms again in the context of cancer.

Withdrawal

During treatment many people describe a sense of wanting or needing to reduce their activities, including the things that normally provide them with pleasure. This can be multifactorial and may accompany a sense of anxiety or feeling overwhelmed when trying to do activities that may normally feel quite manageable, such as catching up with a friend for coffee.

In a cancer context, the physical exhaustion is usually the driver for this, with people wanting to do things but being unable to do so because they are not physically well enough.

Low motivation

As an extension of the physical side effects, people often find that their motivation is low during treatment. This is usually temporary in nature; when people recover, they are normally able to re-engage in what they would normally do, although if they are feeling particularly fatigued they may find it more difficult than usual to motivate themselves. This might change from day to day, with some good days and some bad days. When you physically feel better, you will probably want to do more.

Negative thoughts

Again, this is generally a temporary side effect of being unwell. When people are unwell, most of their energy goes towards getting well again, and it is at these times that people occasionally describe the presence of negative thoughts. They might have some thoughts about whether they will ever be well again. The general process is that when people physically start feeling better their mood improves, and their thoughts return to normal. If such thoughts continue when you are feeling physically well, I would advise that you seek professional help in managing them.

Sense of hopelessness about the future

Again, as above, in the midst of feeling unwell or if people have long admissions in hospital, these kinds of thoughts commonly start to appear on the landscape. The same holds true as for the other negative thoughts: when feeling physically well again these generally subside or become much more manageable.

The other challenge within cancer land around these thoughts is related to the cancer itself. As we have talked about, almost all people who are diagnosed, or have their cancer return, feel worried and think about a potentially limited future, and so in this context it is normal and appropriate to have some of these thoughts present. However, they can be difficult thoughts to manage on your own, and sometimes they are not thoughts that are easy to share with family and friends. For many people, seeing someone to talk about these kinds of thoughts and how you make sense of them can be very helpful.

Changes in the way you feel or interact with other people

In the context of treatment and medications, the way you feel about being around other people might change a little. We will talk about medication effects in Chapter 26 but it is not uncommon for people to feel intolerant of social situations, noises, tastes and general things that would not normally worry them too much. This is usually related to the treatment itself, and subsides when the treatment has finished. But if you feel like this is not the case for you, it is worth discussing with someone.

Many patients work out ways to manage their environment so that they are not exposed to things they know will irritate them while on medication. For instance, if on a particular medication people feel they are unable to manage the noises their kids make, they might go and stay at a relative's place for a couple of days until it has passed. If this is happening for you, and is likely to happen a lot because of the ongoing nature of the treatment, it is definitely worth coming up with some creative solutions to try to reduce the stressors where you can.

Physical changes

This could almost be a chapter in itself when we talk about the impact of the treatments. As we spoke about in the treatment chapters, fatigue, changes in appetite, changes in your body, medication effects and the processes of treatment itself will all impact your body, and in turn your capacity to manage thoughts and emotions. I would encourage you to speak frankly with your team if you are having physical side effects that don't feel like they are well managed, as there are often strategies that might help, and usually if you don't communicate that you are having difficulties people will assume that you are not!

So which is it: depression or cancer treatment?

I suspect this information might not have clarified things as much as you might like. So, I would say that a good rule of thumb for working out what is an effect of treatment and what might be pointing towards something more like depression is to look at timeframes and context.

Do all of the above issues occur when you are sick or feeling physically unwell, and then improve when you are physically feeling better? Or do they linger on, and even when you are feeling physically well do you struggle to manage thoughts and worries, or find it hard to motivate yourself? If it is the latter, it is worth seeking help in managing them.

Do I need medication?

Another common question people ask is whether they need medication. For some people the idea of medication such as antidepressants will seem completely unacceptable, and for others it will seem like the only solution to where they are. For some people medication is definitely the best option, while others will work with their treating team first up to see if they can make some improvements without it.

Also, it is worth noting that antidepressants and anti-anxiety medications can be used for a bunch of different reasons, so if you are on them it might not be for depression. We know that people who take antidepressants experience the best improvements when the medication is paired with other strategies such as therapy and exercise, so it is likely that seeking some help from a therapist will be important.

Will this go away?

Most people I encounter in the cancer setting who are depressed because of their situation, find their depression resolves when they are able to work out ways to manage it. We know that one of the risks for having depression is having been depressed in the past. So, if you have a history of depression or any other mental health concerns, it is likely you will be referred to someone in the context of your cancer treatment, not because we think anything is wrong, but because some work is needed to prevent any further difficulties.

I was really depressed before, but since the cancer it has gone away

This happens too. More commonly than you might expect.

Sometimes, prior to a diagnosis if people are struggling with their mood and managing depression they might be overwhelmed by the process. However when they are diagnosed the focus will change and the 'survival instinct' we have spoken about before comes into play. It doesn't mean the depression won't ever come back, but many people find that their depression feels easier to manage in the future after their cancer experience.

16.

Anxiety

I had never felt anxious before my cancer, but then all of
a sudden I saw the danger and uncertainty everywhere.
The panic felt like it was taking more away from me than
the cancer.

Ahmed, 45 years old

Anxiety is a normal part of life. We all have it, and we all need it. Otherwise we likely wouldn't get out of bed in the mornings. We definitely wouldn't ever do public speaking, or go on a date, or jump out of planes. We need some level of arousal to stop us doing things that are unhelpful or dangerous, but we need some to make sure we do anything at all. The measure of this is about balance, though.

Anxiety can wear lots of hats, and appear in lots of different ways, but in most cases it will appear in our bodies, in our brains or as a combination of both. In our bodies, it can look like difficulty breathing, having a racing heart, feeling tingly in the arms and legs, butterflies in the stomach, or having the urge to go to the toilet. In our brains it tends to be racing thoughts, and often these racing thoughts are about all the things that might possibly go wrong. And for some people, these things come together in unison.

The way I think about it, anxiety largely exists on a continuum, with some people having much more anxiety than is helpful, and some having less. Those who have lots might find themselves worried and overthinking everything they do; they may even feel paralysed by it, and unable to make decisions or even leave the house, seeing danger in every situation that life might present. At the other end of that equation, though, too little means that people are unlikely to complete tasks, or may put themselves in dangerous situations due to feeling disconnected with the systems that are in our bodies to help us navigate the world.

We have already talked about the role of anxiety in managing chemotherapy, and it is likely that these themes will continue to appear through lots of our discussions about cancer in general. In a cancer context there are many reasons why people might be anxious — there is a lot going on that is unfamiliar, there is a threat of danger in our lives, and many of the things that need to be done are inherently quite unpleasant. It makes perfect sense that you might have some feelings of avoidance, worry and wanting to escape, which are some of the key hallmarks of anxiety. Before we get too much into thinking about the anxiety component, I think it is important to explore what underpins much of the anxiety that occurs in this space.

Uncertainty

Such a little word, but such a big impact.

It is likely that before your diagnosis you believed that the world was largely predictable, right? You had planned things, and mostly they worked out. You had been going to work, or maybe had even set yourself up so that you could retire. You had been making plans for yourself, and possibly your family. You might have been working towards a particular goal or plan you had created. Even though you know that bad things happen to people, you had been looking after yourself, or you had told yourself that they wouldn't happen to you.

Does that sound about right? It might sound flippant when I describe it in this way. But I don't mean it to; it is just a description of how many people experience their lives. We need to have distance and separation from an awareness that, actually, most of our worlds are more fragile and unpredictable than we would like to believe. However, for you right now, you see the truth.

Uncertainty is a difficult concept to manage, as it is not something that can be problem-solved or worked with in a way that makes it feel unimportant (which can be how we manage many other difficult aspects of our lives). And this uncertainty is high stakes. The uncertainty around cancer is likely to be very connected with worries about mortality and the future. So trying to dismiss it or the anxiety it drives is unlikely to work very well.

Let's explore the types of anxiety that appear, and how to manage them. (Hint: the answer isn't to get rid of it!)

The types of anxiety that tend to occur in cancer land fit into four main categories:

1. Anxiety about the cancer and treatment itself.
2. Anxiety about finishing treatment or the cancer coming back (we talked about this in Part 2).
3. Anxiety about specific things, like needles or procedures.
4. Anxiety that isn't really about cancer at all.

We've talked a little about number 1 already, and number 2 is covered in a later chapter. For now, we will leave number 3 and come back to it, and number 4 will follow some of the same principals as numbers 1 and 2.

Confused yet?

Anxiety about cancer

Although some of the anxieties around cancer are very specific, there are a few strategies that will work for them, and for many anxieties in general. These concepts are based in the ideas of Acceptance and Commitment Therapy (or ACT).

Simply put, the concepts behind ACT are that the nature of our world is such that we will experience some suffering from time to time, and rather than fighting against this, we work with it. Often our instinct to manage difficult thoughts is to get rid of them and push them out of our minds. But this rarely works: the thoughts generally just end up appearing somewhere else at another time. We have already talked about some of these concepts (see page 34), where we discussed letting your thoughts be present and not getting too caught up in them.

I know this might all sound a bit funny and quite abstract, so let me see if we can wade through it a bit.

Let's go fishing

Imagine that you go fishing (keep in mind that I am not a fishing person so if the details of the analogy are off, I apologize!). Picture yourself standing on a sandy beach next to a little inlet, feet on the ground, maybe even wriggling your toes in the cool sand. You throw out your fishing line and wait to catch something.

You get a bite. The line starts to go tense and you reel in your catch. You are so excited. But then you see what you have pulled in: it's just a little one. You take the hook out and throw it back in.

The thing you can't see from the shore is how many of the fish are little and how many are dinner-sized. So you keep fishing, hoping that you will catch one the right size.

Our brains work in a similar way. There are thoughts being pumped out all the time, over and over again. Some of them are helpful, some of them are unhelpful and some aren't really either. When we are anxious or worried about something, we are likely to keep catching the same thoughts. The ones that tell you how bad everything is, or how likely it might be that something could go wrong in the future. Now of course in cancer land, something has gone wrong, so it makes sense that your brain will be thinking about the possibility of things going wrong in the future. So it's likely you might have more worries than you would have had before. And as we have talked about in previous chapters, trying to get rid of such thoughts rarely works.

So, to manage our worries now we are going to do the same thing you do when you go fishing. When you catch something unhelpful, unhook and throw it back.

I know it sounds strange, but it works. Perhaps it is worth practising right now. Close your eyes, picture yourself standing on that shore, fishing rod in hand, and every time a thought comes in, reel it in (you can picture the words of the thought on a fish if you like) then unhook and throw it back in. Then do the same with the next one. Over and over again until you feel comfortable that the thoughts that come are just little fish that you can manage and deal with.

For these kinds of thoughts it isn't helpful at the moment to look too much at their content, because once you go down that path you will likely find yourself getting all tangled up in them and going down the rabbit hole. As we know, these can go from one little thought to a whole bunch of thoughts very quickly. So, just notice that you have caught them, then unhook and throw them back.

Anxiety about specific things

> I had always been able to avoid hospitals and needles, but now I have no choice. Just thinking about the needle makes me feel faint. I would almost consider not having treatment just to make sure I didn't have to have all those needles.
> Dan, 40 years old

Now, I promised we would come back to number 3. Those particular fears or worries about a specific thing are a bit trickier to deal with. Lots of people walking around in the world have phobias about particular things. But unless these things are related to medical care (like needles, blood or procedures) it's probably manageable. For instance, if you have a strong fear of spiders or flying you have probably worked out ways to manage this in your everyday life. But if the thing you are fearful of is something you require for your cancer treatment, like needles, it might be a bit more of a complicated situation.

Generally, the way of managing phobias psychologically is to do something called graded exposure. This works by teaching strategies to manage the anxiety in gradual steps, so that when you are faced with the thing you're most scared of, you can develop ways to manage the anxiety around it. Like all anxieties, avoiding the thing you are fearful of is likely to make the anxiety worse, so it is important to get some support around this, particularly as, in this situation, if you are fearful of medical things it is unlikely you will be able to avoid them. Importantly, if you are worried, make sure you let your medical team know you are phobic of particular things — it will allow them to work with you to try to manage it. If they do not know you are scared, they won't be able to help!

Specific phobias are not usually something you can manage on your own. My advice is to go and talk to someone at your hospital about how to manage this.

So, when you notice that those anxious thoughts are coming up, go fishing and see what happens if you catch them and throw them back. It doesn't change how many fish are in the sea, and it doesn't change how often you pull out the little ones, but it might change how often you get really tangled up with the thoughts that do appear.

Because, right now, the anxiety and those little fish are helpful. It's just your brain trying to do its job. If there weren't any fish in the ocean it would be a much bigger problem.

17.

Sleep

I imagined I would be so exhausted from treatment that I would pass out as soon as my head hit the pillow. Instead, I was lying awake until all hours, thinking about everything that was going on.
Jonathon, 40 years old

Sleep is a tricky thing — it is of course vitally important for our capacity to function in the world, but it is one of the first things that becomes out of sync when we get stressed or our world is in chaos.

For some people, sleep is a constant battle: they either find they can't get to sleep, or if they do, they will wake in the night and be unable to get back to sleep, having their brains churning out worry after worry. Others will go to sleep at night and not remember a thing about it until the next morning when they wake up refreshed.

Most people at some time have had a period in their lives when they are not sleeping very well, or feeling like the sleep they are getting is not very good. How we are sleeping can be a symptom of the other things in our lives; work stress, relationship stress or other life events can impact sleeping patterns. In addition to this, sleep patterns can become quite habitual quite quickly, so if you wake up at 3 a.m. a couple of nights in a row, quite reliably you will wake up just before that time each night. So, it makes sense that in the middle of the cancer stuff you might not sleep as well as you normally would.

There can be some patterns in sleep disturbance at this time. Firstly, whenever people get a diagnosis or any kind of big news it is likely that sleep will be a bit messed up for at least a couple of days. So the night before scan results, or the night before you start a new treatment, most people will describe not sleeping very well. This is to be expected, and is okay. What we tend to worry about much more is when sleep has a prolonged change over time, separate to any big events or medication impacts.

There are some other reasons for sleep disturbance at this time (and I am not going to go into too much detail here; this is more about you being aware of them). These things are generally related to treatment and medications. Some chemotherapies can cause some sleep disturbance, as can drugs called steroids (which I will talk about a little later on) that many people get with their chemotherapy. They work well for helping to manage a bunch of things including nausea and pain, but one of the side effects is that they can wreak havoc with your sleep. If you are on these medications and are not able to sleep, it is worth talking with your treating team to see if there are things they can do to help manage this.

Worry and sleep

The other thing that can disturb your sleep can be anxiety or worry — which makes some sense in the context of cancer, right?

What can happen is that people are keeping themselves very busy all day with appointments, or sometimes just other distractions to keep them from thinking about things. But our brains being our brains, they will want to think about things anyway, and the best time to do that is in the middle of the night when there isn't much else going on. So it isn't uncommon for those thoughts that you work very hard all day to keep at bay to appear in the small hours of the morning.

There are some things that will feel helpful to work through and think about. These are often things that have a concrete solution, such as working out some of the financial details, or who is going to pick up the kids on Tuesday. So you might wake up and think about these things, but you will often be able to fall back to sleep once you have worked out a strategy. However, the bigger, more nebulous things might be a bit harder to shift. These are the thoughts about uncertainty, like what is going to happen next, or what happens if the cancer comes back. The difficulty with these kinds of thoughts is that it is hard to get to an answer that will feel okay and manageable. Even if you spend time thinking about them, they are likely to keep whirring around in your brain anyway (particularly at 3 a.m.).

So, what can help with all of this?

Be sleep conscious

You know all of those things that people talk about for managing sleep, like having baths before bed, drinking chamomile tea, not watching television (or any other screen!) and only using your bedroom for sleep and sex? They are all really important things.

The reason people talk about them a lot is that they tend to be helpful! For instance, many people get into the habit of waking up in the middle of the night and then reading on their phone to go back to sleep; however, what happens is that the phone stimulates your brain, so it has the completely opposite effect. A good rule of thumb is that if you are going to do something to help you get back to sleep, it needs to be something that slows down your brain rather than speeds it up: reading a really boring book (something that is an actual book, not an electronic one), listening to some music and tuning in to a particular instrument, counting your breaths, doing a sleep meditation (there are thousands of these about, and generally in any meditation app there will be a sleep meditation available) or using your mind to create a picture or a scene (revisiting a holiday location you have visited, or replaying in your mind a favourite movie scene).

If these things aren't working, get up and walk around the house for a bit, or go and do something really boring. I have had patients over the years do things like the ironing, or counting the small tiles on the kitchen bench. The main thing is that these things help slow your brain down, and get you to think about something other than what is keeping you awake. Your brain will naturally try to keep pulling you back towards your worries. That's okay; when that happens, consciously shift your thoughts back to thinking about the other task you want your brain to do.

Sometimes doing something with the thoughts is helpful

Many people give themselves permission to spend fifteen minutes or so during the day to think about all the difficult thoughts that come into their minds — counterintuitively, this can improve things. So, if there are lots of things buzzing around in your mind, set yourself some time where you won't be interrupted (not before bed!) and write down all the things that are worrying you. This works best if you use a pen and paper, as when you see things written down, your mind immediately starts to process them differently to the way it does when they are whirring around in your brain. Then, at the end of the fifteen minutes, pack the list away and go and do something nice. Over the next 24 hours, when things come into your mind that you need to worry about, write them down and tell your mind that you will worry about them in that next fifteen-minute window (including if they come up in the middle of the night). Over time, what tends to happen is that the same worries keep popping up again and again, and your brain learns to recognize them and process them differently.

Accept that not sleeping is okay

One of the things that brings people undone isn't the not sleeping, it's the *anxiety* about not being able to sleep. Not sleeping when you want to sleep is akin to slow torture: the more you think about not sleeping, the more anxious you become and then the likelihood of sleeping becomes even smaller.

One of the ways to manage this — and this advice is particularly true for people who have medical reasons why they aren't sleeping — is to be okay with not sleeping. Let me explain more. The worst thing that happens from you not sleeping is that you haven't slept. Now sure, you might get a bit grumpy or be tired in the afternoon, but nothing bad is likely to happen. If you have many days of no sleep at all this can be problematic (and if this is happening you should definitely tell your team about it) but most people have a few nights of disrupted sleep and then the system will correct itself.

It is not only worth being okay about not sleeping, but it's a good idea to have a plan of what to do if this happens. Lying in bed ruminating about not sleeping when you know you are unlikely to (as a result, for example, of medication effects rather than worries) is not going to be very productive — so have a plan. For instance, on the nights you take steroids save some movies to watch, or a new book you have been looking forward to. Anecdotally, most people find that when they stop worrying about not sleeping, it improves a lot. I will add a caveat by saying that some people find sleep a struggle all the time, regardless of the cancer. If you are always a terrible sleeper, it isn't likely this will improve with the cancer and all the challenges that come with it (I'll be very happy if it does!). If this is the case for you, then the idea that not sleeping is okay is even more important.

Sleeping tablets generally are not helpful

The drugs that work as sleeping tablets feel really nice for our brains, and so very quickly the drug that worked really well one night will work less well the next night, and before you know it you need three tablets to do the same job as one.

For this reason, medical professionals are often reluctant to prescribe sleeping tablets for ongoing use. If you've been having lots of difficulties, they can work well to get your sleep back on track, which is usually for a night or a couple of nights; or if you are taking a medication that will seriously impact your sleep you might be given something to counteract its effects. But using them longer term might become problematic.

Routine is one of the biggest predictors in how well you sleep

Getting up at the same time each day, exercising, not napping during the day and going to bed at the same time each night all make a huge difference to how well you sleep. Sometimes when on treatment people find their sleep gets a bit all over the place, which is okay in the short term, but keeping routine and structure (which we have talked about a lot during the book) is one of the best predictors of sleeping well. It's worth sitting down and thinking about how you can plan to make sure things look as predictable and structured as possible.

18.

Appetite

When I was told I was having chemo I was hoping I would lose some weight. Instead, I couldn't stop eating because of the steroids. It was like my body was a teenager all over again. I just couldn't get enough food.

Jarryd, 35 years old

It stands to reason that appetite might be disturbed in the context of all the cancer stuff. Just like sleep, our appetite can be easily disrupted by emotional changes (think about what happened to your chocolate intake last time something stressful happened in your life!) as well as changes in our physical self.

Following the information of being diagnosed, or perhaps finding out that things are not going well, almost everyone notices a change in their appetite. Usually in this context people don't feel like eating at all and their stomachs feel nauseated and upset. Some, though, find that they will eat much more, sometimes as a distraction from whatever is going on for them. However, much of the time when there is some kind of a plan, or some clarity about what is happening, appetite will start to return to normal.

Of course, a caveat to this is when the tumour itself is causing the difficulties with eating — which is sometimes the case with tumours that are situated in the head and neck or gastrointestinal tract. If this is the cause of your difficulties, it is best to work with the multidisciplinary team to help develop some strategies in managing your symptoms. If you are experiencing these concerns, you will likely find yourself becoming frustrated and despondent by the impact of not being able to eat.

Eating is one of our most social activities and often forms much of our connection and engagement with our family and friends. Feeling you are not able to engage in this way can be overwhelming and isolating. So, if you are likely to be unable to eat for extended periods of time it is perhaps worth thinking of ways you can continue to engage in social activities that don't involve food.

It is likely that in the course of your treatment you will experience some disturbance in appetite and might lose interest in food. This is generally temporary and could be caused by a bunch of different things — for instance, chemotherapy effects, radiotherapy (if to areas that are sensitive to this), pain killer effects or infections. If this is the case your team will probably give you some advice about the specific things that might help (we will also talk about these a little below).

I hadn't eaten anything for weeks after my transplant — not properly anyway, and then I just started having these intense cravings for a cheeseburger. I hadn't eaten meat for twenty years!
Narelle, 50 years old

Psychologically, eating, or specifically how much we eat, can be a really complex thing. Everyone reading this is likely to have had periods in their lives where they may have eaten too much or too little and made changes to manage it. For some people when life becomes difficult for some reason, the amount they eat can become a way of managing the associated stress.

The challenge in the cancer context is that often things that happen to people (for instance, treatment) might mean that they don't want to eat for fear of feeling unwell. So they might not eat, which is likely to lead to them feeling more unwell, and so the cycle continues. Within the cancer context people also might feel as if they don't have much agency or control, and so food can become the thing that helps manage the sense of uncertainty.

If you are finding it difficult to eat, some of these tips might help.

- *Eat little meals.* If you don't feel like eating and are faced with a giant pile of food, you are likely to feel overwhelmed and not each much of anything.

- *Eat food you like.* I get it: people often offer very helpful and caring advice about what to eat when you are sick. However, in my experience these suggestions are often things that don't taste great. If you are struggling to eat, you probably aren't going to want to eat something you don't like, particularly something that turns your stomach at the very thought of it.

- *Eat the food that suits what you need at the time.* If you feel nauseous then sometimes bland foods are the best bet (like plain crackers or toast), but if you have a filthy taste in your mouth after a medication you might need something that tastes stronger. Some of my patients swear by things like licorice, curry, or salt and vinegar chips to try to cover the taste. If you have mouth ulcers, soft food will be much easier on you.

- *Sometimes chemo can give you weird cravings.* For whatever reason, chemotherapy can often mean that people want specific foods, and these might be things you don't normally eat. Just go with it — listen to your body; it will tell you what you need.

- *Don't eat the things you love around chemotherapy time.* Our brain makes fantastic connections between food and feeling unwell so on the days that you are having chemo, or the days after if you still feel unwell, it is a good plan to not eat the foods you like as you might find you end up liking them much less afterwards.

Eating too much

Sometimes people experience the opposite concern, where the drugs they are on make them eat way too much. This is generally the culprit of steroids. If you just have a dose of steroids with each cycle of treatment it probably won't be too much of a problem, but for people who might be on them for a long time (like patients who have a haematological problem or sometimes for people with brain tumours) you might find that your appetite, and as a consequence your weight, becomes difficult to manage. Just as with no appetite, this is normally temporary, although weight gained can sometimes take some time to come back off after treatment has finished.

There are some things to help this while you are on the medications.

- *As much as possible, try to keep eating as you normally would.* This is likely to be pretty hard as your body is going to tell you to eat a lot, and probably not very healthy things. But simple things like trying to keep to the same mealtimes, limiting your snacks and keeping yourself busy might help.
- *Focus when you are eating.* Often, people eat without too much focus or thought. If you are eating too much, focusing on your eating can help. For instance, something as simple as counting how many times you chew something before you swallow, or putting your fork down between each mouthful, will help slow things down a bit and you are likely to be more aware of how much you are eating.
- *Don't have food in the house that you don't want to eat.* Having a house full of chocolate and snacks when you are taking steroids is a recipe for disaster. If you know you are going to be snacking constantly, think about some things that are okay to snack on frequently. A dietitian is a good person to chat with for some suggestions to help manage this.
- *Find some things to do that aren't eating.* People on steroids often report that all they think about is eating. It generally helps to have some other activities to do for distraction, as well as to give pleasure and meaning. Exercising has the dual benefit of regulating your eating and burning off some of the effects of the steroids themselves.

19.

Fatigue and exercise

It was like no tiredness I had ever felt before. The energy had just drained out of me and I found myself unable to do even the most simple of tasks.

Sarah, 47 years old

It seems strange, perhaps, to have fatigue and exercise together in a chapter. However, in cancer land these things go together much more commonly than you might imagine.

Fatigue

Fatigue can be a very common side effect of many of the treatments for cancer, as well as the cancer itself. Like many side effects the severity can vary from person to person, but most people will experience at least some fatigue as they move through their treatments.

The fatigue that people describe is different to just being tired or needing to sleep. One of my patients once described the notion that the energy would just drain out of her, seemingly without warning, and she would be unable to do anything to stop it. The fatigue that comes from treatment is in some ways different to the fatigue that might come from tumours themselves. We will look at a couple of different strategies to manage both of these aspects of fatigue. The exercise part of this becomes relevant when we start talking about managing the treatment-related fatigue elements of cancer (which is generally what people struggle with the most!).

Many patients report that following treatment it can take time for their energy levels to start to return to what they were like pre-treatment. This can be really disappointing for people who have assumed that as soon as they stop treatment, their energy will start to come back to normal. Instead, it may be that the initial pattern is a reasonably fast return to about 80 per cent of your previous capacity, but then the remaining 20 per cent might take quite a lot longer. This is, of course, assuming a pretty standard treatment course with no complications; if you had lots of long hospital admissions or a prolonged time of inactivity it might take much longer.

A little like the analogy of eating an elephant, the key to managing this is to do small pieces at a time. Rather than pushing yourself to get to the amount of activity you feel that you should be doing, take small steps and do what you can manage. One of the biggest challenges isn't anything to do with physical changes at all: usually the thing that brings people undone is the frustration that comes from not being able to do what they expect to be able to do. So in lots of ways, rather than managing the fatigue, it is about managing the frustration, being kind to yourself and evaluating your expectations about what you think you want to achieve.

Using the units of energy in your day to do the things that feel important

One of the challenges of fatigue is that it can feel as if you are limited in what you can do. When fatigue is due to the cancer — this could be when you are first diagnosed or if you have disease which is difficult to control with treatment — you may find there is some variation in what you can do and when, with some days feeling a little better than others.

Let's assume you have 100 units of energy in a day and you have to spend those energy units across all the things you have to do. This includes things like having a shower, going to the bathroom, having conversations with the neighbours, watching television, eating and so on. Some of these things happen every day, and some of them aren't particularly pleasant but quite necessary. However, with the units you have left you have some choice about how to use them. It might be that spending time with people feels really exhausting, but then at the same time it is good exhaustion, with you feeling quite connected and nourished afterwards. There might, however, be other situations where you find yourself spending time doing something that leaves you feeling really drained and unsatisfied. If this is happening, perhaps it is worth asking yourself how you want to use your units of energy for the day, and what feels the most important. Like I said, there will always be things that take energy that aren't particularly pleasurable, but it's all about balancing the limited energy that you have and making sure you are using at least some of it for things that feel like they are really worthwhile. (Keep in mind that in the midst of all of this, you might find that the things that felt really important before all of this might feel quite different now.)

Another way of managing those units of energy is to save up activities that are stimulating but don't take so much energy — for instance, doing a crossword, reading a book, or spending some time learning something you are interested in -- for days when you're particularly fatigued. There is an energy unit cost for these things, too, but it's likely they are much more manageable on the days you are really feeling fatigued than some of the other activities you might do.

Adjust your expectations

One of the biggest frustrations around fatigue often comes with the knowledge that you are unable to do the things you could do before. If your life has changed in a dramatic way and the things you were able to do before aren't possible at the moment, of course you will be frustrated and sad and maybe even angry (or probably a selection of at least a hundred other emotions that might appear). This is completely okay, and it's also okay to take some time to process these feelings and work out what you want to do with them. But, if every time you try to do something, you get smashed across the head by the reality that you can't do that thing anymore, you will probably feel pretty miserable.

Instead, set goals and expectations that feel reasonable. For instance, you might normally be able to sit quite comfortably and read really complex books — *War and Peace* comes to mind. But now every time you open the book you feel yourself getting frustrated and overwhelmed because you can't follow it. Fatigue can be like having a rubber balloon in your mind, moving around and making it really hard to focus and concentrate. So instead of picking up *War and Peace*, then beating yourself up because you can't concentrate, perhaps find something less complex to read. Or maybe say to yourself, 'I know I can only focus for fifteen minutes, so that's how long I am going to read for.' You can even set a timer if you like. This won't be the case forever, but for now it will be much easier to manage if you are able to set tasks and expectations that are manageable for where you are.

Exercise and move your body

Remember on page 45 I said there was some irony involved in all of this? Well, as it turns out, the best way of managing treatment-related fatigue is to do some exercise. This is, of course, the cruellest of ironies, as for almost all my patients who are fatigued, the most difficult thing they have to do is get up and get moving. But all of the evidence now tells us what has been anecdotally reported by my patients for years: when they are up and moving, doing some exercise each day and being present and active in the world, their fatigue feels more manageable. Now, this is much more relevant for treatment-related fatigue rather than for fatigue that comes directly from a cancer itself, although some of my patients also tell me that doing some exercise and being out in the world helps manage their cancer fatigue as well. The mechanisms of this are probably much more complex than I understand them to be, but the less you do, the less you'll want to do, and so the cycle continues. Fatigue thrives on this cycle.

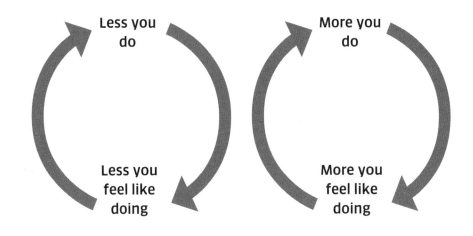

Exercising despite the fatigue

People who are experiencing treatment-related fatigue and take to their beds, not engaging in any movement, reliably tell me that their fatigue is much, much worse than those who are active during their treatment. The guidelines around managing treatment-related fatigue recommend 150 minutes of moderate intensity exercise or 75 minutes of vigorous exercise a week as well as a couple of sessions of resistance work.

> I just couldn't imagine exercising when I felt so exhausted —
> but once I started, I did actually notice the difference.
> Raoul, 50 years old

The main thing when thinking about exercise is to look at how you make it sustainable. Are you a morning person? Because if you aren't I am willing to bet it's almost completely unlikely you will be up at 5 a.m. in the dark exercising. Do you absolutely hate the gym? Then is making a plan to go there every day going to work? Work out what you would like to do, what you can manage, and how you think about it. If you frame exercise as another part of your treatment it might make it more palatable. For instance, I am willing to bet that you don't love chemo but you still keep turning up for it because you feel it is helping you. Perhaps there is some merit in thinking about exercising to manage fatigue in the same way — it is something that might not feel 100 per cent pleasant, but it is going to help you in the long run (and for most of my patients, they feel immediately better after doing something).

Pacing yourself

Now, I know I have just told you to do a bunch of stuff. The key, though, is do things at a reasonable pace over a reasonable period of time. Sometimes as human beings we aren't great at this, right? Think back to the last time you decided you were going to do an exercise program. You probably did loads in the first few days, but then really quickly became exhausted and stopped doing anything (don't worry, this has happened to everyone). This process becomes even more pronounced in the cancer space, when people generally have less capacity for this stuff overall (i.e. fewer units of energy in the day) so it's all about taking it slow and steady, testing the waters and building up to things slowly rather than jumping in with both feet, smashing yourself for a day or two and then being in bed for the rest of the week.

Tell other people what's happening

Sometimes when you tell people you are fatigued or tired, they might think to themselves (or they might verbalize to you), 'Oh yeah, I'm really tired too.' Fatigue is quite a common experience in our existence, however cancer fatigue generally looks quite different. Of course, if you tell those around that you are feeling fatigued they are likely to think about their experience of what it means to feel like that, and they may expect this to be a temporary thing that will be fixed by having a nap or a good night's sleep. This will generally add to any frustration you already have, so in anticipation of that, it is probably worth describing it in a different way: many people say 'unwell' although it depends if for you that feels like a good fit. But using different language means they are likely to engage with you differently around it, and might be able to better understand what you need from them.

As we talked about in Chapter 11, it's a good idea to give the people around you very specific instructions about what you need them to do for you (which might be to leave you alone!). If you don't feel comfortable in expressing these things, it might be worth chatting with someone else who is close to you, to see if they are able to do it for you. This works particularly well if it is about setting expectations for people around how long they might be able to visit for, what you have energy and motivation to do, and how you can communicate your needs to them when you are feeling really fatigued.

Do the things that feel important

I feel it is worth highlighting this one a little bit more. With limited energy, the energy that you expend becomes a much more precious commodity. It's a little like money. If you happen to have millions and millions of dollars in the bank, the cost of the groceries or the petrol doesn't really matter very much. But if you only have $20 in the bank, then those same things and the costs of them starts to feel very different. So imagine if with that $20 someone buys a pot plant, or a tub of car polish — I am guessing you might be pretty grumpy about it. The energy piece works a bit the same: if you end up spending time on things that don't feel important or aren't the right thing for you in that moment, you are likely to feel really grumpy and irritable. This is likely to be particularly true if you are doing things that other people think will be important to you. So think about what you want to do, work out a way to make it feel manageable (even if this means breaking it down into much smaller pieces than you would normally do), and follow through on it. It doesn't fix the fact that you are feeling fatigued, but it is likely to help make you feel much more content, which in turn is likely to make the fatigue feel more manageable.

20.

Body image

Looking in the mirror, the person looking back at me wasn't
the right person, or at least the person I saw in my mind.
Ruben, 19 years old

There is a pretty good chance that some strange things have happened to
your body in all of this. You will have been touched and poked in ways that
are likely to have felt very intrusive in lots of different ways. In addition to
this, you have probably experienced changes in the way your body looks
and functions. These might range from feeling that you are more fatigued
than you have been in the past, to more dramatic things like having had
surgeries that have changed the way your body works.

For almost all patients these changes can feel really confronting and
significant, but can be dismissed or cast aside in the context of knowing
that they are to help manage your cancer. I have heard people say lots of
times that they feel completely uncomfortable in their body, but will just as
quickly say they feel so grateful that the surgery was done so that they can
live. My sense is that these things are not mutually exclusive. It is reasonable

to be grateful and overwhelmed by the knowledge that as a result of intervention you are okay, but at the same time to be able to grieve the loss of your body as you knew it in the past. If you had a car accident and lost your leg you wouldn't expect to wake up and be grateful that it had happened — it would take time and grief, and some sadness and maybe even some anger before you would be able to reconcile the new sense of you and what it means for your body/life going forward. Your cancer experience is similar, and it is likely you won't immediately make sense of it. In fact, it is often after you've had some time to process things that you will have the space to make sense of what any temporary or permanent changes might mean going forward.

The idea of 'normal'

Many people I meet describe really clearly the sense of disconnect between their idea of their 'normal' body and their post-cancer body. Sometimes this might be around function; for instance, feeling that it doesn't work in the same way it previously did. Or it might be that the impact of the treatment has left you feeling deconditioned, and you are asking your body to do things that feel really difficult after a long time of not doing them. Or it might be that when you look in the mirror you don't recognize the person looking back at you (this can be quite common for people who have had surgery to their face) or when you look at your arm or your leg it doesn't feel like your own any more. All of these scenarios are challenging and difficult to try to make sense of.

Many people find their instinct is to avoid thinking about the changes that have happened. They might not be able to bear to look at the scars that have arrived, or similarly may not be able to even think about touching the bits of their body that have changed. Conversely, it may be that people become completely obsessed with the part that has changed, and may find themselves touching it constantly and being acutely aware of even tiny changes that might happen. You may find yourself at one end of this spectrum or you may be somewhere in the middle where you are able to look at and touch the scar but still feel deeply uncomfortable about the changes, or a combination of these things.

It is rare not to have any of these concerns in even a small way. And it makes sense that this is difficult: you have been used to your body looking the same way your entire life, and now all of a sudden it is different. It probably looks different, and usually (at least temporarily) it will feel a little bit different. This takes time to adjust to and make sense of. Initially, people may report being aware of the changes, but then as time goes on they notice them less. I suspect this is caused by a combination of things — over time things probably improve physically, but it seems there is another large part where your mind and brain come to adjust to the changes and work out a way to manage them better.

Managing the changes

It sounds obvious, but how you are struggling with the changes somewhat predicts what you do to manage them.

If you find yourself, for example, constantly touching and being present to your scar, it makes sense that the thing to do is probably make a really strong effort to do things that make you less likely to be present to it. So when you are thinking about it and wanting to touch it, rather than doing that, just notice that is what you are doing and reassure yourself that it is a normal response to want to touch it. But also notice what is happening for you: what happens if you don't touch it? Do you become anxious and uncomfortable? Do your thoughts speed up? Do you start to panic? It's likely that some of the thoughts that come up will be pretty strong around this, and connecting with the scar physically may help to allay these thoughts. The difficulty with this, of course, is that the more you touch it, the more those anxious feelings get pushed away, and the more challenging managing that anxiety can become. So, almost paradoxically, the way to manage the need to constantly be present to the scar is to learn to sit with the anxiety that comes with it. We talked about how to sit with and manage anxiety in Chapter 16, so perhaps it is worth going back and revisiting this if you are struggling with it.

Managing avoidance

The flipside of this is avoidance. If you are avoiding looking at or touching the changed parts of your body, it might help to think about this like a relationship that you need to work on. You have seen your body in the same way for so long; now that it has changed you need to spend time getting to know how things are different and working out ways to reconnect with your body.

Usually, the first step is actually giving yourself permission and time to look at and touch the part of your body that has changed. This is probably going to be hard to do. So like most things that are hard, break it up into smaller steps rather than just jumping in. Are there some steps you can take that will help make it feel more manageable? What are the thoughts that come up around doing it? Here is an example of the steps you might come up with.

> **Step 1:** Look at the area while it is covered with a gown, blanket or clothes.
> **Step 2:** Look at the area while just covered with a dressing.
> **Step 3:** Touch around the area while it is covered.
> **Step 4:** Look at the area for a short time while the nurse is changing the dressing.
> **Step 5:** Look at the area for longer while the nurse is changing the dressing.
> **Step 6:** Help the nurse change the dressing.
> **Step 7:** Look at the area without a dressing on while the nurse isn't around.
> **Step 8:** Change the dressing without the nurse.

The process might be slightly different if you have had surgery resulting in changes to the way you manage your body functions, such as the formation of a stoma. Generally, in the first couple of days post-surgery people feel unable to look at and examine the stoma bag (as an example) or think about how it might work, and usually allow the nurses to do all the care of this. However, as the days pass and as the nurses encourage them to do some of the care themselves, they will generally be able to start looking at and examining the stoma. Almost out of necessity (as being able to manage a stoma can be the determining factor if someone is able to leave hospital or not), after several days people are generally doing most of the care for themselves. Now, it is important to point out that there are few people who do this out of curiosity or want; more often it is about the reality of knowing that in order to continue to have the life they would like to have, they must learn how to manage it. It may, however, take quite a bit longer for them to accept the situation they have found themselves in, and they might struggle with the ongoing process of having to think about, and be present to, the stoma. Over time, however, people do tend to at least come to accept the changes, even if they would still like things to be the way they had been before all of this started.

Other changes

> It sounds strange, but it was easier when I had no hair. At least then people knew that I was sick, and would be nice to me. Now, it's like all of the things that I am struggling with are invisible.
>
> Adrienne, 55 years old

Some of the changes that occur may be much more subtle — changes in your energy levels, or the way your sexual function works. These are things that generally no one can see, which in itself can make these things harder to manage. If people can't see the difficulties, then it's likely they will assume that all is okay, and as a result they might not have very much tolerance for or understanding of what those things mean. This can be quite challenging when it comes to what people expect you to be able to do, particularly in a work or relationship context.

If this is coming up for you it's important that you work out what you need, and then come up with a way to communicate this to the people around you. Remember, if they can't see it they are not likely to be able to help you manage it. I'll talk about this more in the next chapter.

21.

Relationships and sexuality

I wanted to feel close to him, but he was so worried about hurting me and about my body that I felt lonelier than ever, even though I knew he was doing it to care for me.
Jana, 45 years old

It makes perfect sense that some of the things about your relationship might look different in the context of all of this cancer stuff. You might find you become closer and more connected to your partner and the collective sense of managing the cancer might be an important shared experience. Conversely, the experience can be alienating for one or both partners, and you may find that, instead of feeling connected by it, it acts as a wedge between you. Either way, there are likely to be times when you're on a slightly different page to your partner (but hopefully still in the same book!) and how you communicate is important so both of you feel heard and understood.

The biggest challenge in relationships at this time is often communication (yes, I do realize how clichéd that sounds!). It can work both ways. People aren't talking enough about the difficult stuff yet both will have almost the same worries in their minds; alternatively they communicate too much, with the cancer and planning around the cancer becoming the entire focus of their conversations and discussions.

Often, if I get two or more members of a family or a couple in the room, they will both tell me almost identical versions of the same worries or concerns, but will be reluctant to talk with their partner about them for fear of upsetting them. Sometimes the most powerful thing you can do to manage these worries is to name them — pretty reliably, if you are worried about something, your partner probably will be too, and giving it a name and recognizing it then gives you something to work with. There is a pretty good chance that once you have it out in the open you will be much more able to work out how you as a couple plan to handle it. It also means that it is something you can verbalize as opposed to something that is just rattling around in your head.

The other challenge is talking too much about it, so that almost all of your planning and thinking becomes about the cancer. There will of course be times when talking about the cancer all the time is likely to happen, and might even feel helpful; for instance, when you need to make big decisions or if you have had some unexpected news. But much of the time spent during the whole cancer experience is about routine and just getting through the day to day. So if all of your conversation with your partner is about cancer, it's likely it will become miserable for both of you pretty quickly.

Even though it might feel hard to do in the midst of everything, continuing to do all the things in your relationship that make you feel good is helpful, whether that is going out and doing things together, snuggling up on the couch watching a movie or exercising together. If you can't do the things you normally do because of the cancer or the treatment, it is worth discussing other ways you can find to still connect with each other.

When there is lots of other stuff going on, our relationships can be the first things that get neglected. So being really proactive about what you want and need from your relationship, as well as working out what your partner wants or needs, is an important part of this whole cancer thing. However, if you were having difficulties in your relationship prior to the cancer arriving you might find some temporary improvement at the time of diagnosis; but then it is likely that under the stress of treatment and all the things that come from that, those difficulties become evident once again. Some take this as a given and accept that their relationship will continue to be poor, while for others the cancer and sense of time pressure may mean they decide to put lots of energy and effort into trying to improve things. Either way, you might find that the way you feel about your relationship (and other relationships in your life) is different just because of the cancer's presence, and as such the way you think about and behave in the relationship might look really different. If you are struggling with this stuff, it is probably worth consulting professional help, either as a couple or individually, as it is likely that in the midst of all this you will have less emotional capacity to manage any complex relationship issues. It may even be that you decide to deal with anything that comes up after the treatment is finished, when you might have more emotional space to make sense of it.

Sexuality and intimacy

Another challenge couples can find at this time is around sexuality and sexual intimacy. I am going to be straight up about this: most of my patients who are on treatment don't really feel like having sex. Their bodies are likely to feel different, and often they will have much less energy to engage in their normal sexual behaviour. However, at the completion of treatment they can sometimes feel ready to re-engage in sexual activity yet are not feeling comfortable with the bodily changes treatment may have delivered. This can cause tensions and difficulties within relationships if the assumption is that, following treatment, things will just 'go back to normal' and the sexual behaviours you engaged in pre-treatment become the norm once more. The two main difficulties that people can encounter are physical issues and psychological issues.

Physical issues

Physical issues come about as a result of a change in your body or sexual functioning during treatment. This can include surgery or treatment focused on the genitals or abdomen, meaning you might experience some changes in your body which make having sex different or more difficult than before. This can also include changes to hormone levels, which might mean less lubrication or changes in your sex drive; for some men it can mean there are changes to erectile function. For many of the physical changes there will be strategies to manage them, or ways you can discover to work around them. However, this can be a big adaptation and challenge for both you and your partner to make sense of what this new post-cancer sexual engagement might look like.

Psychological issues

The other side of the equation is the psychological aspect of our sexuality, or what we think and feel about our sexual selves. The physical and psychological often go hand in hand and, unlike the physical, the psychological after-effects of cancer can be subtler and harder to fix.

Many people spend lots of energy and attention on the physical fixes of what is happening (and often there can be some tools that will work) but might not put so much emphasis on the psychological aspects. The psychological aspects of difficulties in sexuality and intimacy can be varied and sometimes hard to pin down, even for the people experiencing them. Following such a massive ordeal, and sometimes changes to the way your body might look and feel, it makes sense there would be some lingering effects on how you process and think about yourself in a sexual way.

The psychological effects can be categorized into a few groups (although this is by no means extensive):

- *Feeling uncomfortable in your own body.* It makes sense that if there have been lots of changes to the way your body feels or how it functions it will take time to adapt. It often happens that over time you'll feel more able to manage these changes yourself, but will continue to feel uncomfortable about someone else being present to these changes.

- *Pain.* Pain, as we talked about earlier, can be a really tricky character. It is not uncommon for people who have experienced some pain as a result of sex to then be fearful of that pain happening again. When this occurs it may be that you want to avoid having sex, or any intimacy at all.
- *Worries about performance.* For some people the medications or procedures they have had mean that their physical sexual function has changed. This can mean they become worried or anxious about the impact of these changes, which ends up impacting the performance itself.
- *Relationship concerns.* The nature of your relationship, or even your relationship to sex might have changed through all of this. It may mean that you are evaluating what the relationship means, or what you want it to look like going forward. This becomes really tricky when communication breaks down, and might mean both people in the partnership are uncertain of what is happening with the other.

Returning to sex

> I was so disconnected from my body it was hard to know
> when it felt okay to be sexual again. I hadn't thought about
> it for so long, and bringing that part of myself back into my
> attention felt quite alien.
> Tara, 45 years old

Like many parts of managing this stuff, sometimes the simplest option can be the best. First up, take away the expectation that you are going to jump straight back into having sex and that it will immediately feel exactly the same as it had before. You have likely changed and your body will have changed too, so allow yourself to become comfortable with the fact that, at least in the short term, sex might feel different.

Then — and this may seem like a controversial statement — remember that sex and intimacy isn't just about penetration and it isn't just about orgasm. It's about doing things that feel good. And right now, the thing that might feel good could be not having penetrative sex; it might be holding hands and cuddling. There are lots and lots of programs around to help couples connect on the things that feel good, rather than feeling as if you need to get to a goal of a particular type of sexual act. However, it may be that you and your partner just take a step back and allow yourselves to channel your teenage selves: spend time exploring your body and their body, just because it feels nice rather than because penetration or orgasm is the goal. There are lots of really pleasant things couples can do together that will feel incredibly intimate and bring you closer to each other. It may be that penetration happens at some point, but the important thing is to take the time you need to feel comfortable. However — and I can't stress this enough — you need to be open and transparent with your partner about where you are and what you need. It will always go spectacularly badly if you definitely don't feel ready to have sex but you don't tell your partner, who assumes that you are. These are tricky but really important conversations to have so that you can work together on what you can do to manage this. Even after these conversations, if your partner is pressuring you or expecting that you will be able to have sex regardless, it might be that these difficulties are representative of other things, and getting support is likely to be helpful.

22.

Working

I didn't quite know how to manage the demands of work when I got sick. It had always been my priority, then all of a sudden it didn't feel as important, but I knew that when the cancer passed I would need to go back to it, so I had to make sure that I kept doing a good job.
Joseph, 60 years old

One of the questions I get asked most often is about working during all parts of the cancer process: during treatment, when treatment is finished, and what to do when the work you were doing might not feel the same anymore.

The answer to any of these questions is often a bit nebulous and unhelpful like 'It depends'. The reality is that there are many factors that can determine your capacity to work as you move through the cancer space.

At diagnosis

When a diagnosis comes as a shock it makes sense to stop doing everything until you have a plan. Then you can make decisions about what to do next. Depending on how your situation has developed it might be that there is a delay between diagnosis and treatment, or you might be told you will need to start treatment straight away. Obviously, if you are going to start treatment immediately, you will likely be in a situation where you need to take leave from work (even if you don't want to). Often this can mean you will need to be in hospital (in the instance of acute leukaemia, for example), so working needs to be put on hold as much for practical as for psychological reasons.

However, if you are someone who has had a long period of time between diagnosis and the start of treatment, this decision might be less clear. Some people might clearly decide they don't want to be in a situation where they need to think about work at a time when they are thinking about the cancer stuff and trying to navigate lots of appointments and tests. For others, even though they might not be focusing as well as they did in the past, the structure of going to work could provide some comfort and purpose while waiting to get more information about the plan for treatment and what might come next. This is entirely a personal choice and depends on many factors:

- *How physically well you are.* If you have been diagnosed with something there is a reasonable chance you might be unwell or on medications that could impact your performance at work.
- *How much leave you have.* Many people try to save leave until they absolutely need to take it.
- *How much time there is between things.* If you are spending almost all of your days at the hospital or at appointments, it might feel more stressful to try to juggle work as well.
- *A sense of whether you need to wrap things up.* Many people end up taking a considerable amount of time off work when they are having treatment, so sometimes there is a sense that people need to 'sort things out' at work before they are going to be away, such as doing a handover to colleagues.

- *You work for yourself.* This can be much more complex in terms of being able to have time off, still have cash coming in and contingency planning for what you are going to do with the business over the next little while.

Whatever you decide, it needs to work for you and what you need at that moment in time. Work out what feels helpful for you; the distraction of work might feel right, or you might not have any inclination or motivation to work at all.

During treatment

Many people who commence treatment will be convinced they'll be able to work the whole way through, with maybe a couple of days off here and there. And it's not to say that they won't, but it's important to set realistic expectations about what the next part of the experience will look like.

Chemotherapy

Most people having intensive intravenous chemotherapy struggle to maintain a normal working structure in the midst of treatment. However, it might be that working part-time or working from home allows you to still manage some work. Employers are often more accommodating than you might expect, and will tend to want to work with you to allow you to do what works best for you. As we talked about in Chapter 5 on chemotherapy, the first cycle is often the most difficult psychologically and will generally feel the most unpredictable, so making decisions about work prior to this cycle can be quite difficult. However, once this cycle is done and you know what to expect, it might be that you can speak with your manager and let them know what you are likely to need. If you are on a three-weekly cycle, you might realistically only be able to work for a week, or a week and a half in each cycle. Most people generally overestimate their capacity, so it is better to start small and, if you are able to, do more, rather than the other way around.

It might be that you think you won't be able to work at all, but then find yourself going stir crazy at home a couple of cycles into treatment. If this is the case, it might be worth thinking about what you need at that time. Although, it is also worth thinking about whether there might be other things you could use to fill your time than simply working.

Radiotherapy

With radiotherapy you might physically feel okay until towards the end of treatment, so working could feel completely manageable. However, the challenge in juggling work and radiotherapy is about practicalities: for instance, needing to be at the hospital at a certain time each day, which, depending on your role, can be challenging. That said, usually treatment centres will do what they can to accommodate people so if you need to have treatment before or after work they might be able to come up with some solutions to help you manage it.

Surgery

Surgery will generally require you to have time off. When you meet with your surgeon they will be able to give you an idea of how much time you will likely have in hospital, as well as how much recovery you will need to take after you have been discharged.

For many big surgeries it might be that you are told you will be out of action for at least six weeks after the procedure. It's generally assumed that you won't be able to do any work during that time.

After treatment

As soon as they end treatment, some people are already thinking about getting back to work as soon as possible. There can be some challenges with this, in that it will likely take some time to physically recover from whatever you have just been through. But as we talked about in the section on finishing treatment (see page 69), it is likely that, emotionally, things will catch up with you a bit after that last treatment.

It's important to take time to process this and try to make sense of things. Don't just jump into the next thing, like getting back to work straight away. It's also important that, if you have been away from work for a while, you go back at a pace that is manageable and sustainable. For most people it isn't manageable to go straight from not working at all to being back at work full-time, and will require some gradual return plans, for example starting with two or three half-days per week and gradually increasing back to full-time hours. It is much better to underestimate how much you might be able to manage than to jump straight back into it and then be so exhausted at the end of the first week that you need to take another two weeks off!

Not being able to return to your previous role

There are some situations in which people are unable to return to their previous roles. Sometimes this can be due to managing the challenges of the physical demands of the work; or perhaps, as a result of a surgery or intervention, you are unable to do the same role again.

Companies are usually quite accommodating where possible in returning people to roles, and it may be that they are able to work out a slightly different role you can return to. If not, though, it may mean you will have to explore potential options moving forward, or even look at reskilling, which might feel like a very difficult thing to manage in the context of the cancer experience. If this is the case, it is a good idea to not feel that you need to make perfect decisions at once. Perhaps it is worth dipping your toes into studying something new and starting something very small rather than jumping straight into an intense course or program that you might not feel equipped to manage so soon after finishing cancer treatment. There might also be some external agencies that could help you connect with ideas/ strategies about what you might like to do next. Sometimes making use of career counselling or vocational support is a good idea, as counsellors can be quite realistic about what you might need to go forward.

If you don't want to go back to what you were doing

Sometimes after treatment the idea of going back to the job you were doing previously may just feel wrong. It might be that you can't imagine going back into a busy or stressful job, or that you feel your values have changed and so the job you were doing is no longer a good fit. It might be that you don't know what you want to do, but you know you don't want to return to your previous job. However, just as with any period following a big life event, it is best to let things settle a bit before you make any really big decisions. Perhaps going back to your role is unsustainable in the long-term, but in the short-term going back part-time or gradually returning will allow you some time and space to think about what you want to do next.

Generally speaking, it is always easier to get involved with new things when you are doing something else, so you might find the balance of working in your old role while studying or making some plans about your next thing could be a good fit. Also, you have just had a lot of change in your life, and in all likelihood the thing that feels like a great idea now will still feel the same in three months' time if it is the right one. So allow yourself some time to let things settle before you make any really big decisions, and make a plan before you do anything.

23.

Being present

People just kept telling me that I needed to be mindful, and that it would sort everything out. I kept picturing needing to sit cross-legged on a mat for hours and being Zen. It was helpful for me to know that it didn't need to be like that to be helpful.

Thandie, 45 years old

There has been a massive groundswell in both psychology circles and society in general about the role of mindfulness meditation in the past years. For most of us, the very word meditation is likely to conjure some images which will either feel pleasant or unpleasant depending on your past experiences of it.

There is significant evidence around the role of mindfulness and meditation in the management of all sorts of psychological distress and difficulties with mood and anxiety. In cancer, mindfulness has been shown to reduce psychological symptoms. So, it would be remiss of me to talk about managing psychological stuff in the context of cancer and not talk about it, right?

First up, I just want to point out that there are loads of ways to be mindful and to meditate. Some of those may be in a really structured way like going to a class, listening to a guided process or allocating a specific period of time to do the practice. For some people this will work really well, and meditating in a structured and routine way will make it feel more manageable. However, for just as many people the practice can be shorter, opportunistic and in a way that feels like it fits with their world, for instance when they are walking, cooking or even listening to music.

There can often be pressure for people to feel like they need to conform to a particular type of practice or that it won't work if they don't do it for long enough. But in my experience, any opportunity to be present and take yourself a little out of the worries and thoughts about the future and uncertainty is likely to help, even for a moment.

Some of the best ways to get present are very simple. In fact, for my money, usually the simplest ways are the best and the things you are more likely to stick with. There are loads of exercises for grounding and being present but the ones I like the most are the ones that simply and easily connect you with where you are — where you reassure yourself that right here in this moment 'I am okay' — or where you connect with your breathing or the outside world (such as things that you can hear or smell at that moment). These are easy to do, you can do them anywhere and no one is likely to know you are doing them. They work really well when you are feeling caught up in loads of thoughts or when the thoughts about the future start to feel overwhelming.

You can also do really easy mindfulness while you are doing other things: for instance, when you are listening to music, try tuning in to just one instrument (drums work well); listen to the sound of your feet hitting the ground when you walk; count your steps between two places; or pay attention to the way you are eating. These things also tend to work really well when you find you have thoughts or worries that have caught you a bit, or even if you just want to bring yourself back to being more present to what you are doing. Our world is full of distractions, so sometimes having time to be properly present is a really powerful thing.

There are also more advanced things to do. You might really like doing some visualized meditation, where you picture a scene or image in your mind, then move through or be present to the image in your mind. This can be quite helpful if you have times when you are really unwell and unable to do the things you might normally do to help you manage. You can also use visualization to help you process or think differently about your situation.

There are also many breathing and body meditations that get you to focus on your breathing or on sensations in different parts of your body. These can work really well at times when you don't feel connected with what is happening in your body, but I would advise some caution around this. If you have difficulties breathing because of your cancer you could find that bringing attention to this may exacerbate your anxiety. If this is the case, perhaps it might be better to focus on some of the things we spoke about above. If you're doing an exercise called a body scan (this will be in most mindfulness smartphone apps) at the time you're asked to focus in on the part of your body that is problematic, focus on something else instead. For instance, if you are having lots of pain and discomfort in your spine, then when asked to focus on your back, maybe focus in on your little toes, even wriggling them about and noticing that sensation instead.

Wandering focus

Many people who start doing any of these strategies might be shocked by just how little time they can spend being focused before their brain wanders off and starts thinking about other things. Guess what? You are normal!

One of the most helpful jobs our brain does is to think for us. And it does it a lot, so the idea that your brain will completely disconnect and stop thinking just because you want to focus on the noise the birds are making in the backyard is a bit unrealistic. What is likely to happen is that you will start being mindful or meditating, and think you are doing okay, and then 20 or 30 seconds later (this does improve with practice) a thought, or even a series of thoughts, may show up. This is okay; just notice those things coming into your mind then bring your attention back to whatever you were doing previously. I have never met anyone who is able to do this without any thoughts ever appearing, but you might find that the more that you practise, the more focused time you will have where thoughts aren't popping up so much.

Simple ways to get started

I have listed some simple activities that you can do below. Give them a try, and if one doesn't work for you, try another until you find something that feels like a nice fit for you (this can be a little bit like finding a comfortable pair of shoes ... it's trial and error).

- *Slow down your breathing.* Breathe in as far as you can for five seconds and then breathe out as far as you can for five seconds. Do this ten times. Counting while you breathe gives your brain a job and means you can be more focused. Try to keep your breathing calm, and focus on slowing it down and moving the air into your belly rather than high in your chest.
- *While you are walking, notice your footsteps.* What noise do they make? Are they heavy or light? What does the bottom of your foot feel like as it meets the ground? How many steps do you take between street lights or the distance between two roads?
- *When you are eating, slow yourself down.* Notice what happens in your mouth when you first put the food in. What does it feel like on your tongue or your teeth? Try to chew each mouthful ten times before you swallow. Make sure you swallow everything before you put more food in your mouth.
- *Notice five things you can hear right now.* Are there noises in the room, or if you are outside what is around you? Are the sounds far away or close? What are the noises that are so faint you can barely hear them?
- *Close your eyes and think about your favourite place to go on holiday.* Notice all of the things around you. What are three things

you can smell, taste or touch? What is behind you? If you had to notice a tiny detail in the picture to show to someone else, what would it be?

- *Listen to some music.* Now tune in to the drum beat, and only listen out for that. Then, in the next song, try to just listen for another instrument.

If you are finding it difficult to do these things on your own, as I mentioned earlier there are loads of apps that will give you some options to do all the kinds of things we have talked about. And a silly-sounding tip: if the adult meditations are not working for you try the kids' versions. They are usually much shorter, easier to do, and for the most part more fun! Many of my adult patients have found this to be a good plan if they are struggling to get their meditation in.

24.

Being grateful

Sometimes I just wake up in the morning and think to myself:
I have another day, how wonderful is that!
Vicki, 44 years old

The idea of being grateful when diagnosed with something pretty horrible doesn't seem to make much sense, but it's something that can make a huge different to your perception of how well or badly things are going. The idea of being grateful is definitely not a new one, and it may be that you are actively doing things to recognize and acknowledge the good things in your life and not just the difficult things. The idea of bringing gratitude into daily practice has of late become much more prevalent, with lots of studies showing that engagement with regular recognition of things we are grateful helps us manage depression, anxiety and stress much better.

So what does this look like? Well, generally it is a very simple thing to do: just be present to the things around you that are pleasant, or nice, or that you feel glad to have around you. For some people this starts in the morning when they wake up, and they might name some of the things that are good! It doesn't need to be as dramatic as the example at the start of this chapter; instead, it can be things like, 'I am grateful for a comfortable bed, and that I can be so warm when it is cold outside'. It can be simple things during the day, for instance being grateful for tasty food to eat, or for the sun on your shoulders.

Many people find that writing these things down is particularly effective. Looking at the list of helpful things in your life is likely to be a very tangible way to connect and be present to these things.

Lots of my patients find this happens quite naturally as a result of their cancer experience; they find they are much more tuned into the good things in life, and value the ways these things add to their experience rather than just passing them by.

Why is this helpful?

Sometimes in the midst of all of this cancer stuff it is easy to get really caught up in the things that are not going well. It's easy to catch all the unhelpful thoughts and all the ways that the cancer is impacting your life. You might be too sick to do the things you like to do that give meaning and purpose to your world. But taking some time out to acknowledge and be present to little pieces of your world that are nice and that you're thankful for is a simple way to remember that there are some okay bits in all of this.

25.

Managing other people

If I have one more person tell me that I just need to be positive, or that it will all be okay, I think I might scream. I know they're well meaning, but it drives me mad. They don't have any idea of where I'm at, and them talking like that makes it really hard for me to tell them.

Louise, 39 years old

As we have talked about through the book, one of the trickiest parts of this whole experience is managing other people's expectations and responses to you. Almost everyone will want to be helpful when they hear the news that you have been diagnosed with something, but it may be that they have no idea what might actually be helpful. This can be when things like 'just be positive' or 'don't worry about that' might appear. As we have already established, it's expected that you might worry more about the future than you have in the past, or you may feel you need to talk about things you haven't talked about before. Some people around you might find it really difficult to manage this.

Many patients report sadness when someone in their world is not as supportive as they had hoped. This might be for a whole bunch of reasons, but most of the time it means people feel disappointed that they haven't been able to access the support they need.

On the other side of the coin, it may be that people you haven't been close to, or weren't expecting much from, reach out to you. These people might be the ones who at this time can give you the support you need, or just know what to do. Often they have had an experience of something difficult in their lives and can relate to what might be helpful for you.

If you find that people aren't supporting you in the way you need, perhaps it is worthwhile speaking with them and spelling out what you need. You can give a direction like 'It would really help me if you could get me some bread from the shops as I am exhausted' or 'I don't need you to feel like you have answers for what I am going through, I just want you to listen to me.' They may then be better able to give you what you need.

However, there might be some people who just don't get it regardless of how often you tell them. Many people decide that, during treatment and making sense of all of this, they don't have the energy to try to make other people understand. This is also true for the people in your world who are really distressed by your situation (even when you are feeling okay). Many of my patients make a choice to spend time with people who are able to deal with what is happening, as they don't feel they have the energy to support those who aren't coping as well. This doesn't mean it will feel like this forever, but it's about working out what will help you right now.

The other time when people find it difficult to manage others' reactions are when things change medically. Many patients take time after they find out news of their cancer returning, or if things aren't going well, before they tell other people. This can be based around knowing that the people around them are likely to become distressed so they might need to feel they have processed the information before they speak with other people about it. It can also be a good idea to make sure you feel you have enough information to share for it to be helpful — for instance, knowing what the plan is, or what you think about something before you try and explain it to other people. If not, it might be that you get bombarded with questions you don't have answers for, which is likely to just add to how overwhelmed you might feel.

26.

Pain

In those moments when I was in pain, I would have done anything to get out of it. It was at those times when I truly thought that dying would be a better option so I wouldn't have to think about it anymore.

Emma, 34 years old

Pain is a tricky concept.

Most people have experienced some pain in their life — even if it's a headache or a stomach ache. There are some people who manage to live with and tolerate incredible amounts of pain in their everyday lives, and somehow become accustomed to it and manage it while being able to maintain a semblance of a normal life. However, for others any pain can become completely overwhelming and they can find themselves unable to do the tasks and activities they would normally like to do or manage. Most of us have some ideas around being fearful of pain, and if I ask people about what they worry about in the future in the context of their cancer, many people identify pain.

Pain is usually your body letting you know that something is wrong. Sometimes it can be a small thing — like sleeping at a funny angle and waking up with a sore neck. Or it could signal something much more serious like the growth of a cancer pushing on a nerve which causes pain. Most of us are pretty tuned in to what happens in our bodies when pain is around; it is a pretty difficult thing to manage, and often people become quite distressed by its presence. When you have pain, particularly significant pain, it's likely you will find it hard to concentrate, may be grumpier and more irritable, and thinking about anything other than the pain might be really hard. When I sit in a room across from anyone who is in pain, they tend to shift around a lot like they can't get comfortable, and they generally struggle to focus on whatever we are talking about.

It's important that we distinguish between acute pain and chronic pain. An acute pain is one that comes on suddenly and is generally quite strong in nature (although not always) and is usually time limited. Chronic pain, on the other hand, tends to have a longer course and is the kind of pain that might be less amenable to quick solutions. So, in a cancer sense an acute pain may occur due to the effects of a tumour or an illness, whereas a more chronic pain might result from surgery, where the impact is that a part of your body doesn't work in the same way and there is a pain response.

Managing pain

I am not going to get into the nitty gritty of managing pain too much here (there are many people in your team who will be much better able to do this) but it might be helpful to chat about some of the ways that working with your pain can help manage it.

Recognize that you are in pain

This sounds obvious, right! However, pain can masquerade as many different things. Most people will be able to identify that a really sharp stabbing pain is in fact pain, but may not recognize some of the other signs, like discomfort or not being able to settle. These can be the early signs of pain prior to the pain becoming more severe, so being connected with these other sensations (which are also pain) can help manage the overall pain.

So, think about when you have been in pain — did you shift around a lot, were unable to get comfortable, or have a vague area of discomfort somewhere? If you think of these things as pain as well, it can help keep your pain under control.

Keep on top of the pain

One of the things about pain (particularly cancer pain) is that it usually behaves pretty predictably. What I mean by that is that it's likely to keep showing up until something happens to change the presence of it (like treatment or surgery). So, in those times when it is present, people usually take medications to manage it and then hopefully it will go away; then when it comes back they will take more medication. But when the pain is fully present it takes time for the medications to work, so you will likely have periods of high pain, which is difficult and exhausting. So a better strategy is to take medications when you notice those early signs, such as discomfort, that we spoke about above, and work with your doctor on a regular regime of medication, like taking your medications every six or eight hours so the pain doesn't have a chance to come back to full strength.

Take your medications

Lots of people are anxious about taking medications for pain and this is reasonable as quite strong pain medications are usually prescribed for cancer pain. However, in the cancer space it is incredibly rare for people to experience addiction and dependence on these medications, and if this were to be the case, your team would have strategies to help you manage it. I can count on one hand the number of people who have had difficulties coming off their pain medications, and in most cases the opposite is true: the pain subsides and people very happily stop using their medications.

Follow the advice of your doctors for managing drug side effects

Let's face it, many of the drugs used to manage pain come with some side effects. For most people, the side effects feel okay in the context of the trade-off of pain management. However, there are likely ways of staying on top of the side effects so that they don't become problematic.

The main side effects come from the medications slowing down your gastrointestinal system, making you constipated — usually people on these medications will also be given other medications to counteract this. And the other main side effect is feeling fuzzy or cloudy in the mind — this tends to be worst when you first start taking the medications, with improvement over time. Although there usually aren't any medications to manage this, you might be able to manage it with strategies such as finding less challenging tasks than you would normally do (reading a magazine instead of a book might be easier, for example) or finding strategies that help to get your brain working better, like going for a walk outside or being mindful.

Use other strategies to help manage your pain

There are plenty of things people do to help manage their pain. These include physical strategies such as exercise, yoga, acupuncture, massage or other touch therapies. There are also some psychological strategies that might help — some people find meditation for pain is really helpful, or conversely that using distraction to think about other things, rather than focusing on the pain, can help. As long as these strategies feel helpful for you, it doesn't matter which one you use — but it may take a little bit of trial and error to work out which is the right one for you.

Notice which thoughts accompany your pain

It sounds strange perhaps, but your thoughts can have a huge impact on your experience of pain. Most of the time there are two experiences of pain: the physical one and the psychological one. The physical experience is the actual sensation of pain which is happening in your body — such as a sore knee. And the psychological experience is any thoughts you have about this, for instance, 'Great, I've woken up with a sore knee again and I won't be able to do anything today.' Most people find it difficult to think about anything else if they have significant pain, but it might be worth noticing what some of the thoughts are that accompany the pain, and what they are telling you. They are often quite difficult thoughts and this can mean you might find them difficult to examine and work with; but identifying the thoughts that accompany your pain can also mean you are better able to deal with the physical experience of it. This can particularly be the case if you have more of a chronic pain picture and need to make sense of what it might look like to live with the pain ongoing.

Different kinds of pain

For some people, the first sign of cancer being present might be pain. Conversely, the experience of having the cancer managed may bring some pain (such as post-surgery). It is likely there will be some differences for you in what this pain might look like — many of my patients are able to distinguish between the different types of pain (cancer pain vs being unwell pain vs surgical pain) and will develop strategies that work to manage these various types of pain.

Just as we spoke about sleep and anxiety in Chapter 17, sometimes being able to work with the pain in the context of knowing that it is likely to be present will actually mean that you may struggle less with the idea of the pain and what it means to have it present in your life. As I mentioned earlier, with very acute and significant pain this will not likely be helpful, but with ongoing pain that will continue to be present in your world, it can be really helpful to work on strategies to allow the thoughts and impacts of pain to feel manageable rather than overwhelming.

Summary of Part 4
The psychology part: How can you manage all of this?

Managing cancer and everything that comes with it can be psychologically really challenging, and it might be that as you move through this you experience feelings or emotions you have not previously felt. One of the most helpful things in managing this is to allow yourself to experience these as they come, rather than fighting against them. This is hard stuff, and your brain needs to work out what to do with it.

Here are some key things to help get you through.

Communicate

The people around you will think they know what you need, but it may be they are completely off the mark. Unless you tell them what is happening for you, or what you need from them, they will probably get it wrong.

When you are off treatment and start looking well again, the people around you might forget that you still need support — it is okay to tell them that you need them to ask you how you are, help out with things, and for them to understand that you are different because of what has happened.

Check in with yourself about how you are coping

This is a long process and most people will at some stage feel like they are coping less well, feeling anxious, not sleeping, or maybe even feeling depressed and hopeless. This is all okay and expected, but there is help around to get you through it. Check in with yourself, and seek help as needed.

Be present and connect with gratitude

There will be lots of things that are tough and uncertain as you move through the cancer stuff. However, if you are able to stay present and in the current moment, as well as thinking of things that help you feel grateful and connected, you are more likely to be able to tolerate all the other things that are going on.

Make choices that work for you

Being a cancer patient comes with lots of pressure, with almost everyone having ideas about what you should or shouldn't do. You are the person going through this, and it is okay to work out what you need and block out the rest. All of the information that will come to you will be delivered with good intention — it may just be that for you, in that moment, it won't be a good fit. There is no right or wrong way to manage this, and you will find the way that best works for you — and it's okay if it doesn't match what other people might want for you.

Some final thoughts

People tell me all the time how brave and exceptional I am.
They look at me in disbelief and think that I am wonderful
for being able to do all of this. I smile, but I know it's rubbish.
What other choice do I have? I just need to get it done, and
live my life at the same time.
Ruby, 19 years old

So, we have reached the end of the book. Hopefully by now you have managed to pick up some helpful tips and strategies to help you manage through the experience of living with cancer, or caring for someone who is living with cancer. As I promised at the beginning, there are no shortcuts or things that will make this easy, but my hope is that some of the things we have talked about may just make the day to day of it a little bit easier to bear.

We have talked through the emotional processes of being diagnosed and some of the things that commonly come up for people around treatment. We've also discussed coming off treatment and the worries and anxieties that come up around this for people.

The experience of cancer has likely changed you forever. This isn't necessarily about being morbid or dramatic; but having something arrive in your life that challenges your assumptions about what you think is important, what you value, and what you want the future to be like even in the smallest ways, means it will stick with you for a long time. There aren't many other experiences in life where this occurs. Some people embrace this and find ways to change their world based on what they have learnt, while others might return to a world that looks almost identical to their pre-cancer world, with the impact of the cancer flashing back to them from time to time. Either of these is fine, as is somewhere in the middle.

Hopefully, one of the things you have gained from this book is an awareness that even when difficult things happen, you have the skills and capacity to deal with them. If in the year prior to you getting cancer someone had told you that it would happen, you would have been completely overwhelmed and likely told them there was no way you could manage it. But here we are. It may not always be ideal, or there might be things you would do differently if you had your time again, but the reality is that as human beings we are inherently resilient. Most of my patients tell me they know they don't have a choice in managing any of this, and there comes a comfort from knowing that if this kind of thing happened again, they would manage that too.

You now have the skills for managing into the future. It may be that you have now finished the cancer part and are navigating making sense of what happens next; or you might still be in the midst of it, or it might have come back. Regardless of where you are in life, the skills you have been able to apply to managing your cancer stuff can be applied in other parts of your world.

Even in the worst of times you can work out a way to stay present, connect with people, be kind to yourself, thank your mind and your brain for trying to help you and find even the tiniest of things to be grateful for. And the rest of the time, when things aren't terrible, it's good to find these things too. After all, I am willing to bet that during all this you have become very connected with the things you value and the stuff that is really important.

If after reading this you feel you need some more support there are many avenues for you. If you are being treated in a big hospital they will probably have emotional support services available (either psychology, social work or spiritual/pastoral care) and if you call the switchboard they will be able to point you in the right direction. You might need a referral from your doctor or a nurse, or you may be able to refer yourself. In smaller hospitals these services might not be available, but your GP will be a good source of who to refer you to in the community. Ideally, you would want to see someone who knows about cancer or works with people with health conditions, but most important is to see someone who feels comfortable for you. I have always thought that finding someone to talk to is like finding a good, comfortable pair of shoes: you know pretty quickly if it is a good fit. There are also lots of community resources who can point you in the right direction if you aren't sure where to go to access support.

There are many ways of thinking about this whole cancer piece, and you will find your own story — whether things go well or whether there are times that are fraught with difficulties. The most important part is allowing yourself to feel the things that come to you, see them for what they are, and to remember that there is no perfect way of doing this — you will just do the best that you can.

> I think maybe I have learnt lots of things about myself through all of this. I have learnt that I am a person first, and the cancer is just hanging around. I am a friend, and a good listener. I like to laugh, and play games and be silly. At the end of all of it the cancer will do what it will do, and I am still going to be me.
>
> Maya, 25 years old

Acknowledgments

Firstly, this book and the thoughts within it would not exist without the many people who I have met and worked with over the years who have shared some of their most private and nuanced thoughts about their cancer experience, and the ways they have made sense of it all. I am more than grateful for the work we have done together.

Gareth, Anouska, Karen and the team at Exisle have been incredible to work with. They have given consideration, collaboration and time that has allowed this book to develop. I look forward to more projects together.

I have had the privilege of working with some of the most skilled clinicians in Psycho-Oncology, and in ACT. I cannot fail to mention Nicole Ferrar, Angela Cotroneo, Catherine Adams, Fran Orr, Iris Bartula, Julie Grove, Emma Dickens, Katherine Cameron and Vivek Bhadri, who have all shaped how I think clinically and are also great friends. A special mention to Julie Grove who with incredible patience continues to help me keep the ship on course.

Eileen, Catherine and Michael, and the Executive team at Chris O'Brien Lifehouse — my strength as a clinician has been nurtured by your support, both personally and professionally. To the Allied Health and Psycho-Oncology teams at Lifehouse — I see how hard all of you work, and how much you value the work that you do.

Finally, to do this work, there need to be things outside of it. I have an incredible group of people who make up my world — Gayleen, Renee, Ian, Charlotte and Sue, as well as people who are too many to name, but you know who you are. Renee — I am very glad for you to be my sister, and for our awesome friendship.

And to T. We make lots of choices in life, and one of the most important seems to be who you choose to spend it with. I chose very well indeed.

References

Angiola, J.E. and Bowen, A.M., 2012, 'Quality of life in advanced cancer: An Acceptance and Commitment Therapy view', *The Counselling Psychologist*, 41. 2. 313–35. https://doi.org/10.1177%2F0011000012461955

Beatty, L. et al., 2017, 'A systematic review of psychotherapeutic interventions for women with metastatic breast cancer: Context matters', *Psycho-Oncology*, 27. 1. 34–42. https://10.1002/pon.4462

Butow, P. et al., 1996, 'When the diagnosis is cancer: Patient communication experiences and preferences', *Cancer*, 77. 12. 2630–7. https://doi.org/10.1002/(SICI)1097-0142(19960615)77:12%3C2630::AID-CNCR29%3E3.0.CO;2-S

Ciarrochi, J., Fisher, D. and Lane, L., 2006, 'The link between value motives, value success, and wellbeing among people diagnosed with cancer', *Psycho-Oncology*, 20. 11. 1184–92. https://doi.org/10.1002/pon.1832

Clinical Oncology Society of Australia, 2018, COSA position statement on exercise in cancer care, available online: https://www.cosa.org.au/media/332488/cosa-position-statement-v4-web-final.pdf

Cormie, P. et al., 2018, 'Clinical Oncology Society of Australia position statement on exercise in cancer care', *The Medical Journal of Australia*, 209. 4. 184–7. https://doi.org/10.5694/mja18.00199

Epstein R. and Street R., 2007, 'Patient-centered communication in cancer care: Promoting healing and reducing suffering', National Cancer Institute, NIH Publication No. 07–6225. Bethesda, MD.

Feros, D.L. et al. 2001, 'Acceptance and Commitment Therapy (ACT) for improving the lives of cancer patients: A preliminary study', *Psycho-Oncology*, 22. 2. https://doi.org.au/10.1002/pon.2083.

Greer., S., 2008, 'CBT for emotional distress of people with cancer: Some personal observations', *Psycho-Oncology*, 17. 2. 170–73.

Harris, R., 2007, *The Happiness Trap: Stop struggling, start living*, Exisle Publishing, Dunedin, NZ.

Hayes, S. et al., 2006, 'Acceptance and Commitment Therapy: Model, processes and outcomes', *Behaviour Research and Therapy*, 2006. 44. 1. 1–25. https://doi.org/10.1016/j/brat.2005.06.006

Hulbert-Willliams, N.J., Storey, L. and Wilson, K.G., 2014, 'Psychological interventions for patients with cancer: Psychological flexibility and the potential utility of Acceptance and Commitment Therapy', *European Journal of Cancer Care*, 24. 1. 15–27. https://doi.org/10.1111/ecc.12223

Jacobsen, P. and Jim, H., 2008, 'Psychosocial interventions for anxiety and depression in adult cancer patients: Achievements and challenges', *AC: A Cancer Journal for Clinicians*, 58. 4. 214–30.

Ledesma, D. and Kumano, H., 2008, 'Mindfulness-based stress reduction and cancer: A meta-analysis', *Psycho-Oncology*, 18. 6. 571–9. https://doi.org/10.1002/pon.1400

Linden, W. et al., 2012, 'Anxiety and depression after cancer diagnosis: Prevalence rates by cancer type, gender and age', *Journal of Affective Disorders*, 141. 2–3. 343–51. https://doi.org/10.1016/j.jad.2012.03.025

Maguire, P., 1999, 'Improving communication with cancer patients', *European Journal of Cancer*, 35, 10, 1415–22. https://doi.org/10.1016/S0959-8049(99)00178-1

McBride, C. et al., 2000, 'Psychological impact of diagnosis and risk reduction among cancer survivors', *Psycho-Oncology*, 9. 5. 418–27. https://doi.org/10.1002/1099-1611(200009/10)9:5<418::AID-PON474>3.0.CO;2-E

Mosher, C. et al., 2018, 'Acceptance and Commitment Therapy for symptom interference in metastatic breast cancer patients: A pilot randomized trial', *Supportive Care in Cancer*, 25. 1993–2004.

Osborn, R.L., Demoncada, A.C. and Feuerstein, M., 2006, 'Psychosocial interventions for depression, anxiety and quality of life in cancer survivors: Meta-analyses', *International Journal of Psychiatry in Medicine*, https://doi.org/10.2190/EURN-FV1K-Y3TR-FK0L

Otto, A.K., Szczesny, E.C., Soriano, E.C., Laurenceau, J.-P. and Siegel, S.D., 2016, 'Effects of a randomized gratitude intervention on death-related fear of recurrence in breast cancer survivors', *Health Psychology*, 35 12. 1320–8. http://dx.doi.org/10.1037/hea0000400

Savard, J. et al., 2006, 'Randomized clinical trial on cognitive therapy for depression in women with metastatic breast cancer: Psychological and immunological effects', *Palliative and Supportive Care*, 4. 3. 219–37.

Stanton, A. L., 2012, 'What happens now? Psychosocial care for cancer survivors after medical treatment completion', *Journal of Clinical Oncology*, 30. 11. 1215–1220. DOI: 10.1200/JCO.2011.39.7406

Wood, A.M, Froh, J. and Gerahty, A.W., 2010, 'Gratitude and well-being: A review and theoretical integration', *Clinical Psychology*, 30. 7. 890–905. https://doi.org/10.1016/j.cpr.2010.03.005

INDEX